THE ENDOCRINE PANCREAS AND JUVENILE DIABETES

ADVANCES IN EXPERIMENTAL MEDICINE AND BIOLOGY

Recent Volumes in this Series

Volume 117
STEROID HORMONE RECEPTOR SYSTEMS
Edited by Wendell W. Leavitt and James H. Clark

Volume 118
CELL SUBSTRATES: Their Use in the Production of Vaccines and Other Biologicals
Edited by John C. Petricciani, Hope E. Hopps, and Paul J. Chapple

Volume 119
TREATMENT OF EARLY DIABETES
Edited by Rafael A. Camerini-Davalos and Bernard Hanover

Volume 120A
KININS – II: Biochemistry, Pathophysiology, and Clinical Aspects
Edited by Setsuro Fujii, Hiroshi Moriya, and Tomoji Suzuki

Volume 120B
KININS – II: Systemic Proteases and Cellular Function
Edited by Setsuro Fujii, Hiroshi Moriya, and Tomoji Suzuki

Volume 121A
MACROPHAGES AND LYMPHOCYTES: Nature, Functions, and Interaction, Part A
Edited by Mario R. Escobar and Herman Friedman

Volume 121B
MACROPHAGES AND LYMPHOCYTES: Nature, Functions, and Interaction, Part B
Edited by Mario R. Escobar and Herman Friedman

Volume 122A
PURINE METABOLISM IN MAN – III: Clinical and Theoretical Aspects
Edited by Aurelio Rapado, C. H. M. M. de Bruyn, and R. W. E. Watts

Volume 122B
PURINE METABOLISM IN MAN – III: Biochemical, Immunological, and Cancer Research
Edited by Aurelio Rapado, C. H. M. M. de Bruyn, and R. W. E. Watts

Volume 123
GABA – Biochemistry and CNS Functions
Edited by Paul Mandel and Francis V. DeFeudis

Volume 124
THE ENDOCRINE PANCREAS AND JUVENILE DIABETES
Edited by David M. Klachko, Ralph R. Anderson, Thomas W. Burns, and Harold V. Werner

THE ENDOCRINE PANCREAS AND JUVENILE DIABETES

Edited by

David M. Klachko

Ralph R. Anderson

Thomas W. Burns

and

Harold V. Werner

University of Missouri - Columbia
Columbia, Missouri

PLENUM PRESS • NEW YORK AND LONDON

Library of Congress Cataloging in Publication Data

Midwest Conference on Endocrinology and Metabolism, 13th, University of Missouri, Columbia, 1977.
The endocrine pancreas and juvenile diabetes.

(Advances in experimental medicine and biology; v. 124)
"Proceedings of the Thirteenth Midwest Conference on Endocrinology and Metabolism, held at the University of Missouri, Columbia, Missouri, September 28–30, 1977 and sponsored by the University of Missouri – Columbia, College of Agriculture . . . [et al.]"
Includes bibliographical references and index.
1. Diabetes – Congresses. 2. Pancreas – Secretions – Congresses. 3. Diabetes in children – Congresses. 4. Diabetic angiopathies – Congresses. I. Klachko, David M. II. University of Missouri – Columbia, College of Agriculture. III. Title. IV. Series.
RC660.M53 1977 616.4'62 79-21998

ISBN 978-1-4684-8510-3 ISBN 978-1-4684-8508-0 (eBook)
DOI 10.1007/978-1-4684-8508-0

Proceedings of the Thirteenth Midwest Conference on Endocrinology and Metabolism, held at the University of Missouri, Columbia, Missouri, September 28–30, 1977 and sponsored by:

University of Missouri – Columbia
- College of Agriculture
- Dalton Research Center
- Department of Biochemistry
- Department of Child Health
- Department of Family & Community Medicine
- Department of Medicine
- Department of Pharmacology
- Department of Physiology
- Department of Radiology
- Department of Surgery
- Department of Veterinary Anatomy & Physiology
- Department of Veterinary Medicine & Surgery
- Department of Veterinary Pathology
- Division of Biological Sciences
- Extension Division
- Graduate School
- School of Medicine
- Sinclair Research Farm
- University Assembly Lecture Committee
- Veterinary Medicine Diagnostic Laboratory

Eli Lilly and Company
Mead Johnson Research Center
Ross Laboratories
Upjohn Company
Wyeth Laboratories

Softcover reprint of the hardcover 1st edition 1979

A Division of Plenum Publishing Corporation
227 West 17th Street, New York, N.Y. 10011

Conference Chairmen

RALPH R. ANDERSON, Ph.D., Associate Professor of Dairy Husbandry, UMC

DAVID M. KLACHKO, M.D., Associate Professor of Medicine, UMC

Planning Committee

JOHN D. DAVID, Ph.D., Assistant Professor of Biological Sciences, UMC

C. W. FOLEY, Ph.D., Professor of Veterinary Anatomy-Physiology, UMC

LEONARD R. FORTE, Ph.D., Associate Professor of Pharmacology, UMC

JOHN M. FRANZ, Ph.D., Associate Professor of Biochemistry, UMC

JAMES A. GREEN, Ph.D., Professor of Anatomy, UMC

LAURENCE W. HEDLUND, Ph.D., Assistant Professor of Dairy Husbandry, UMC

MURRAY HEIMBERG, M.D., Ph.D., Professor of Pharmacology and Medicine, UMC

J. ALAN JOHNSON, Ph.D., Assistant Professor of Physiology, UMC

CALVIN W. WOODRUFF, Professor of Child Health, UMC

WARREN L. ZAHLER, Ph.D., Assistant Professor of Biochemistry, UMC

Speakers

ROBERT S. BAR, M.D., Assistant Professor of Medicine, Division of Endocrinology and Metabolism, University of Iowa College of Medicine, Iowa City, Iowa

BURIS R. BOSHELL, M.D., Ruth Lawson Hanson Professor of Medicine; Medical Director, Diabetes Research and Education Hospital, University of Alabama School of Medicine, Birmingham, Alabama

MICHAEL BROWNLEE, M.D., Chief Fellow, Joslin Clinic, Boston, Massachusetts

REX S. CLEMENTS, JR., M.D., Associate Professor of Medicine; Director, Clinical Research Center and Metabolic Research Laboratories, University of Alabama, Birmingham, Alabama

JOHN E. GERICH, M.D., Associate Professor of Medicine and Physiology; Director of Diabetes and Metabolism Research Laboratory, Mayo Medical School, Rochester, Minnesota

RACHMIEL LEVINE, M.D., Executive Medical Director, City of Hope Medical Center, Duarte, California

CHARLES R. PARK, M.D., Professor and Chairman, Department of Physiology, Vanderbilt University School of Medicine, Nashville, Tennessee

ARTHUR H. RUBENSTEIN, M.D., Professor and Associate Chairman, Department of Medicine, University of Chicago, Chicago, Illinois

MARK A. SPERLING, M.D., Associate Professor of Pediatrics; Chief, Pediatric Endocrinology and Metabolism, U.C.L.A. School of Medicine, Harbor General Hospital, Torrance, California

MICHAEL W. STEFFES, M.D., Ph.D., Associate Professor, Department of Laboratory Medicine and Pathology; Medical Director of Clinical Chemistry Laboratory, University of Minnesota Medical School, Minneapolis, Minnesota

JOSEPH R. WILLIAMSON, M.D., Professor of Pathology, Washington University School of Medicine, St. Louis, Missouri

Moderators

THOMAS W. BURNS, M.D., Professor of Medicine and Director, Division of Endocrinology and Metabolism, UMC

RICHARD A. GUTHRIE, M.D., Professor and Chairman, Department of Pediatrics, University of Kansas School of Medicine, Wichita, Kansas

ROBERT C. HARDIN, M.D., Professor of Medicine, University of Iowa, Iowa City, Iowa

MURRAY HEIMBERG, M.D., Ph.D., Professor and Chairman, Department of Pharmacology, UMC

ROBERT L. JACKSON, M.D., Professor of Child Health, UMC

HAROLD V. WERNER, Assistant Professor of Medicine, UMC

Discussants

BREITENBACH, R.P., Division of Biological Sciences, University of Missouri-Columbia

BURNS, T. W., Department of Medicine, University of Missouri-Columbia

DAVIS, J. W., Department of Biochemistry, Saint Louis University, Saint Louis, Missouri

FRANZ, J. M., Department of Biochemistry, University of Missouri-Columbia

GUTHRIE, R., Department of Pediatrics, University of Kansas School of Medicine, Wichita, Kansas

HAIBACH, H., Department of Radiology, University of Missouri-Columbia

HEIMBERG, M., Department of Pharmacology, University of Missouri-Columbia

IVEY, K. J., Department of Medicine, University of Missouri-Columbia

JACKSON, R. L., Department of Child Health, University of Missouri-Columbia

KILO, C., West County Internal Medicine Inc., Saint Louis, Missouri

KLACHKO, D. M., Department of Medicine, University of Missouri-Columbia

PETERSON, C. M., Department of Medical Biochemistry, The Rockefeller University, New York, New York

SANNY, C. G., Department of Biochemistry, College of Osteopathic Medicine and Surgery, Des Moines, Iowa

SHEAR, D. B., Department of Biochemistry, University of Missouri-Columbia

TOWNSEND, J. F., Department of Pathology, University of Missouri-Columbia

VORBECK, M. L., Department of Pathology, University of Missouri-Columbia

WEINSTEIN, I., Department of Pharmacology, University of Missouri-Columbia

WERNER, H. V., Department of Medicine, University of Missouri-Columbia

Preface

Dr. Robert L. Jackson, Professor of Child Health at the University of Missouri-Columbia, decided to retire from clinical practice in 1977 and the Department of Child Health planned a conference in his honor. The Thirteenth Annual Midwest Conference on Endocrinology and Metabolism also was in the planning stages and scheduled for two days in the fall. It seemed appropriate to combine the two into an expanded three-day conference. In view of Dr. Jackson's international reputation in the study and care of children with diabetes mellitus, the conference topic was not difficult to find. Experts in this field were delighted to be asked to speak at a conference in Dr. Jackson's honor. We selected a number of excellent speakers to survey the physiology and pathophysiology of pancreatic hormones and their effects in diabetes mellitus, to discuss current knowledge of the microvascular complications of the disease, and to put it all into the proper historical perspective of where we have been and where we are going. We think the conference achieved its objective to pay meaningful tribute to a distinguished member of the scientific community.

As with any conference, the conversion of the presentations and discussions to the printed page is a long and arduous process. Many manuscripts were completed well after the conference and references often are more recent than the date of the conference. We wish to express our appreciation to all participants in the conference, to the planning committee, to Mrs. Linda Bennett who typed the copy, to Plenum Press for their assistance and, especially, to the sponsors without whom the conference could not have taken place.

Ralph R. Anderson
Thomas W. Burns
David M. Klachko
Harold V. Werner

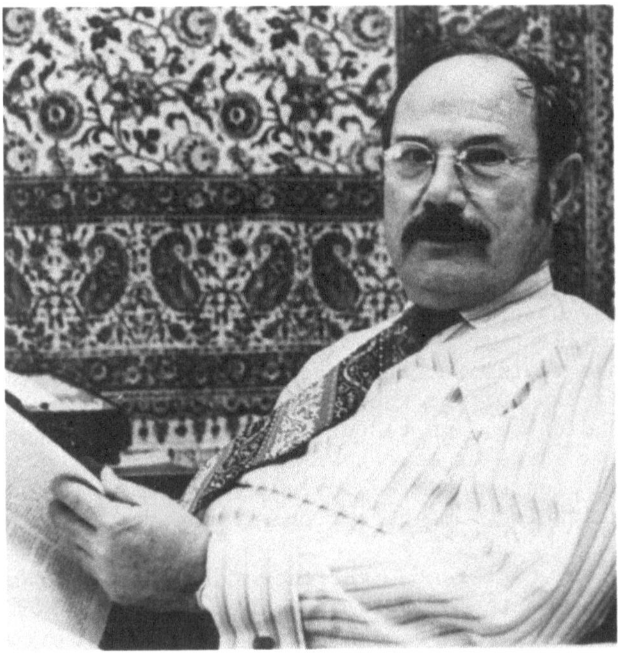

Robert L. Jackson, M.D.

ROBERT LAWRENCE JACKSON

Robert Jackson is a native of Michigan and was born in the town of Clare in the central part of the lower peninsula where he attended the public schools. He received the Bachelor of Science degree from Notre Dame University in 1930. Subsequently, he studied at the University of Michigan and was awarded the M.D. degree. From 1934 to 1937 he was first a rotating intern and then a resident in Pediatrics at the University of Iowa Hospitals, including an exchange residency at the University of Rochester. In the years 1937 to 1954 he remained at the University of Iowa in advancing ranks from Instructor to Professor of Pediatrics. In 1954 he accepted the Chair of Pediatrics at the University of Missouri-Columbia in which capacity he served until 1973. Since then he has remained active as Professor of Pediatrics.

These are but milestones which tell us little about the person whose journey they mark. He is, and was always, a talented physician, teacher, and research scientist whose energy was spent in making better the lives of children, both sick and well. The interesting questions are: What led him to these endeavors? What did he accomplish? Why did he devote himself to these tasks?

The last question, "Why," cannot be answered with certainty because individuals rarely understand themselves so completely and observers never do. Probably what one does in life is a product of opportunity and personality. As will be recounted, Dr. Jackson had an early introduction to biological research and this, judging subsequent events, caught his interest.

An even temperament which has enabled him to succeed arises in part, at least, from certain facets of his character of which four come to mind. First, he has a deep religious faith which is a natural part of his everyday life.

Second, he is truly a "family man." He and Mrs. Jackson have enjoyed many years together and have raised a family which is a constant source of pleasure and support.

Third, he has but one approach to all people. He is a superb clinical scientist and a demanding teacher, but with students, patients, patients' parents, and colleagues, the only interpersonal relationship he understands is friendship. A warm regard for him as a person persists in patients and students for years after their initial contact.

The fourth characteristic is a true love for children -- his own, his patient, or, for that matter, any child. This is the solid base for all his work and is, perhaps, as close as one can come to "why."

How he proceeded into his life work is a bit easier to ascertain. As an undergraduate at Notre Dame he majored in chemistry and as a senior was a laboratory assistant in organic chemistry. It was then that he did his first research which concerned the chemistry of pyridine. While a medical student at Michigan he worked at a community hospital in Ann Arbor, St. Joseph Mercy Hospital, and became involved in investigation into cystinuria and the pharmacological properties of caffeine. Research became a daily part of life as a house officer and soon after he began to focus on two fields in particular -- diabetes and nutrition. In many ways these studies were related, particularly those concerned with the nutritional needs and the growth and development of diabetic children. Dr. Jackson made important contributions in the field of rheumatic heart disease and the prophylaxis of rheumatic fever and in renal disease. However, the major thrust for 40 years has been the management of the juvenile diabetic.

Since the discovery of insulin, the treatment of the child with diabetes has been revolutionized. In the beginning, absolutely nothing was known about what would happen to a diabetic child whose life was prolonged by insulin. Since then, much has been learned and each step of the way has been illuminated by Dr. Jackson. He was influenced by Dr. Julian Boyd who postulated very early that the goal of treatment should be a return to normal physiology, including normal growth and development. Dr. Jackson played a major role in the establishment of norms of growth of well children and demonstrated that these could and should apply to diabetic children. To this end, he conducted nutritional studies and research into the effects of various types of insulin, their combinations, and timing of their use. With his coworkers he demonstrated fully that the diabetic child could achieve a normal life.

Finally, he turned his attention to the question of whether the specific vascular disease of diabetes could be prevented by treatment. This last work has continued to the present day and there is now a widening acceptance of the necessity for careful control of the juvenile diabetic. These would seem to be the outstanding ones among Dr. Jackson's many contributions to medical art and science.

Recognition has come from many places. Invitations to serve on national boards and committees speak for the respect in which he is held, as do many lectures he has been invited to give. He has been honored twice by the American Diabetes Association -- with the Banting Medal and with the first award given for work with diabetic youth.

It is always pleasant to speculate about what an individual might pick from among his accomplishments as the one that pleases him most. It is also an exercise fraught with great chance for error, since none of us can really know another's most private feelings. I would presume, on a long association, to guess that Bob Jackson would choose the many friendships he has among those he has helped -- students, patients, patients' families, and colleagues.

This conference, and this volume arising from it, are a fitting tribute from some of those friends.

Robert C. Hardin

Contents

THE ENDOCRINE PANCREAS, PAST AND PRESENT 1
Rachmiel Levine
Discussion 11

CLINICAL SIGNIFICANCE OF C-PEPTIDE 15
A.H. Rubenstein and B. Gonen
Discussion 21

GLUCAGON: SECRETION AND ACTIONS 29
Mark A. Sperling
Discussion 53

SOMATOSTATIN--ANOTHER PANCREATIC ISLET HORMONE 63
John E. Gerich
Discussion 79

INSULIN RESISTANT SYNDROMES IN HUMANS. 85
Robert S. Bar, Michele Muggeo, and Jesse Roth
Discussion 101

BIOCHEMICAL DERANGEMENTS IN DIABETES MELLITUS. 105
R.S. Clements, Jr.
Discussion 121

BASEMENT MEMBRANES IN MUSCLE CAPILLARIES 133
C. Kilo and J.R. Williamson

BIOCHEMISTRY OF THE BASEMENT MEMBRANE IN DIABETES
MELLITUS 141
Michael Brownlee and Robert G. Spiro

DIABETIC GLOMERULOPATHY: A DYNAMIC PROCESS PRO-
DUCED BY THE DIABETIC ENVIRONMENT. 157
M.W. Steffes, D.M. Brown, and S.M. Mauer

DISCUSSION FOLLOWING TALKS ON MICROVASCULAR COMPLICATIONS OF DIABETES MELLITUS 167

DIABETES MELLITUS CHALLENGES FOR THE FUTURE. 175
B.R. Boshell and B.S. Trippe
Discussion 195

INDEX. 201

THE ENDOCRINE PANCREAS, PAST AND PRESENT

Rachmiel Levine

City of Hope National Medical Center
1500 East Duarte Road
Duarte, CA 91010

Our certain knowledge of the relationship between pancreatic function and diabetes mellitus is roughly 100 years old. However, informed speculation of a possible role played by this gland recurred in the literature periodically from 1787 onward. The story is a fascinating one, full of advances and retreats, faultless logic and foolish errors, but above all serendipity, which finally led to the proven relationship established by Minkowski and Von Mering in 1889.

To understand this tortuous road of discovery it might be useful to review the pioneer attempts at insight into the causes of diabetes beginning with Thomas Willis in 1674. Dr. Willis, you will remember, contributed mightily to the subject by doing the first chemical test in diabetes. He tasted the urine of a severe diabetic and found that it was sweet (Willis, 1674). This was a mighty contribution because very soon after that one could distinguish between diabetes mellitus and diabetes insipidus, meaning a kind of diabetes in which the urine had no taste; it was <u>insipid</u>.

At that time it was not known what substance was responsible for the taste. This was reserved for speculation for the next 100 years and it was another English physician, Matthew Dobson, who advanced the subject by taking the urine of severe diabetics and heating it in a kettle over a fire. The water was boiled off. The residue resembled rock candy (Dobson, 1776). Dobson and Cruikshank then weighed the "candy," and thus began to quantitate degrees of glycosuria.

At that same time, Dr. John Rollo was Surgeon General of the Artillery of the United Kingdom. A captain in the Artillery, Mr.

Meredith, became diabetic and was in a severe clinical phase when Rollo attended him. Rollo had not seen many diabetics but he made a very thorough study of Meredith's case and, with the help of Mr. Cruikshank, he found that the amount of "sugar" in the urine correlated best with the amount of starchy food eaten by Captain Meredith the day before (Rollo, 1797).

Of the most prominent symptoms, polyuria, frequency and loss of weight, the polyuria attracted the greatest attention. Thus, the seat of the disease speculatively became the kidney. The kidneys permitted sugar to escape and, thus, caused the body to waste away. "The flesh melted into the urine." On that basis, Brisbane gave diabetics cantharides, which have a nephrotoxic action (Brisbane, 1773).

The kidney thus became the focus of attention. Rollo, however, drew the conclusion that the central organ in diabetes was the gut, since there was a direct relationship between the amount of "vegetable matter," that is starch-containing foods, and the amount of sugar found in the urine. He argued that it was more reasonable to suppose that the digestive tract of a diabetic may well convert starch into sugar at abnormally rapid rates. The kidney simply excreted the excess. This was a major advance in thinking.

The first mention of the pancreas in diabetes occurred about 1795 in a very interesting paper by a country practitioner, Dr. Cowley (1788). Dr. Cowley published a post mortem report on a patient with diabetes whom he had treated for years. He remarked that the pancreas was almost completely shriveled and full of stones. He drew no etiological deductions from it. The kidney was mentioned as being swollen and pale, the liver as having some fatty transformation.

This report alerted clinicians in England, in Germany, and in France to look for lesions of the pancreas whenever they had a chance to do an autopsy on a diabetic. Occasional scattered reports of pancreatic lesions in diabetics began to appear.

Again, no etiological relationship could be deduced because the knowledge of the role of the pancreas in digestion and metabolism was rudimentary in the first half of the nineteenth century.

About the year 1815 the French chemist, Chevreul, a remarkable person, who lived until the end of the 19th century (aged 104 at his death), demonstrated that the sugar in the urine of diabetics was not cane sugar but glucose or grape sugar (Chevruil, 1815).

In Chevreul's laboratory there worked a young man at that time, a physician who wanted to learn chemical techniques. His name was Apollinaire Bouchardat. Mr. Bouchardat's first paper on diabetes appeared in 1838, and from that point on, at intervals until 1875, there appeared memoirs on diabetes as he gathered experience and data about the disease. The data included blood and urine sugars, uric acid determination, amylase estimations, etc. (Bouchardat, 1852).

He called attention to the frequent occurrence in certain cases of diabetes of high uric acid levels. In his writings he emphasized that not all cases of diabetes were of one type, clinically and/or chemically. He and also Lancereux (1877) began to distinguish between "lean" and "fat" diabetes. The French term is Diabete maigre and Diabete gras. They showed that Diabete maigre, or lean diabetes, was a severe disorder with a very poor prognosis. Diets, opiates, bleeding, etc., gave only fleeting relief. In many of these lean diabetics post mortem revealed severe pancreatic lesions. "The diabetes of the fat" was more common. It was milder clinically and was not associated with weight loss. As a matter of fact, these people tended to be obese. In other words, the division into what we now call "juvenile onset" versus "adult onset" diabetes was made between 1850 and 1875. Bouchardat pointed out that the adult obese diabetic could be helped to survive in good condition. The regimen of value consisted of the reduction of caloric intake especially focused on carbohydrates, loss of weight, and severe physical exercise performed every day of their lives. Gross pancreatic lesions were not found when such diabetics came to autopsy.

The suggestive data that the pancreas may play a role in the genesis of diabetes was not taken seriously by the contemporary authorities in experimental medicine. Claude Bernard, the discoverer of glycogen and of the role of the liver in sugar production, the then acknowledged authority in the field of experimental diabetes, tested the notion of the possible role of pancreatic function in the disease and found it to be a false idea. He (as well as Moritz Schiff in Italy) injected paraffin into the pancreatic ducts of animals. The substance hardened, blocked the ducts, and caused "complete" atrophy of the glands. However, the animals with the atrophic pancreatic glands did not become hyperglycemic (Arnozan and Vaillard, 1884; Bernard, 1856).

Many years later, armed with hindsight, it became evident that the term "complete" atrophy of the pancreas simply meant a 98% atrophy with retention of the endocrine cells, which were, of course, unknown at the time.

The negative experiments and opinions of Bernard and of Schiff were reinforced by pathologists. When pathologists began to gather data on diabetes they could only find pancreatic lesions in a small number of cases. Histological examinations were not yet well developed. Since they did not make the distinction between "lean" and "obese" diabetes, they lumped the data all together and said that pancreatic lesions were present only in a small percentage of cases. Therefore, this could not have any significant etiological meaning for diabetes as a whole (Dieckhoff, 1895).

Meanwhile, in 1869, completely unaware of this controversy, Paul Langerhans was finishing his senior year at the medical school in Berlin and was working in Virchow's Department in pathology. As his graduating dissertation he published his finding of some hitherto undescribed cells in the pancreas of rabbits. They appeared to be either of lymphoid origin or, perhaps, they stemmed from the nervous system. He called them little "heaps of cells," what we now know as the islets (Langerhans, 1869). But when this was published in 1869, it fell to the bottom of the lake of literature like a stone and wasn't heard about for years.

The next time we came to any serious consideration of the pancreas in diabetes was 1889: the decisive work of Minkowski and Von Mering (Mering and Minkowski, 1889; Minkowski, 1893). It is the impression of most people that these workers performed pancreatectomy in dogs because they thought that there was a relationship between the pancreas and diabetes. This is not so. Minkowski himself, in a letter written in 1929, gave the exact details of why he and Von Mering were led to remove the pancreas in dogs in 1889 (Minkowski, 1929).

Minkowski knew the literature on the pancreas and was in accord with M. Bernard that there was not an etiological relationship between the pancreas and diabetes. He was a member of the faculty of the medical school in Strasbourg as assistant to Bernard Naunyn. Naunyn was the most renowned clinical figure in diabetes in Europe at that time. Minkowski was the discoverer of the *beta*-hydroxybutyric acid in diabetic coma. He knew human diabetes thoroughly. The notion relating the pancreas to the disease, however, was not in his mind, since Bernard had "shown" definitely that an atrophic pancreas is compatible with a perfectly normal blood sugar level.

Von Mering working in pharmacology had discovered the glycosuric effect of phlorhizin. Around 1889 he was engaged in the study of fat absorption. He told Minkowski that he was forced to give up this area of research, because it had become important to explore the role played by the pancreas, but he had been told on good authority that it was impossible to do pancreatectomy in the dog and have the animal survive the procedure. The authority quoted was again Claude Bernard.

Minkowski would not easily accept authoritative dicta of this nature. Within several hours of the above conversation, the two colleagues had operated on some dogs and left for the weekend. The surviving depancreatized animals were to be used in studies of fat absorption. It was noted by the animal caretaker that the operated dogs, who were house-trained beforehand, began to urinate frequently and had become very unruly. Minkowski's experience with clinical diabetes led him to test the urine with a copper solution. There was, indeed, intense glycosuria.

The actual discovery of the relation of the pancreas to severe diabetes mellitus was thus serendipitous.

Meanwhile, the concept of internal secretion was already in the air, although the term hormone had not yet been invented. The idea of an internal secretion controlling the blood sugar was not as outlandish as it might have seemed, even a short time before 1890. The internal secretory nature of the pancreas was slowly established by Minkowski (1893), Hedon (Hedon, 1892; Minkowski, 1929), and Laguesse (Laguesse, 1849, 1910).

Minkowski carefully removed the gland, but left one small piece under the skin. Diabetes did not develop. When a few days later, he removed that small piece of tissue diabetes began to develop. Hedon confirmed these experiments *in toto*.

Laguesse was an expert histologist. He resurrected the work of Langerhans, and suggested that the "heaps of cells" were the site of production of the internal secretion. He named them the Islets of Langerhans. Thus, Minkowski's and Hedon's work and Laguesse's findings permitted the conclusion that the islets formed a gland of internal secretion within the body of the pancreas; and that this gland must have something to do with the regulation of the blood sugar. The name "insulin" was proposed for the hypothetical substance since it was produced by islands or insulae (Meyer, 1909).

There followed a remarkable series of papers by the Italian pathologist and histologist, Diamare (1899, 1924), and the American anatomists, Lane (1907) and Bensley (1911-12). These workers pointed out that the Islands of Langerhans consisted of more than one cell type. This provided the first hint that perhaps we were dealing with more than one internal secretion.

The approaches via histology were soon succeeded by extraction and chemical purification, and later still, pharmacological and physiological attempts at mechanisms of actions.

Soon after the successful use of insulin in man, it was noted by Murlin (Kimball and Murlin, 1923) and by Buerger (Buerger and Kramer, 1928) that when insulin was given intravenously the blood sugar first rose significantly before it began to fall. Buerger and Murlin suggested that there may be another substance in the pancreatic extracts containing insulin. They called that substance glucagon, an agonist for glucose. This had about the same immediate scientific fate as Langerhans' finding of the cells; the suggestion was ignored for a long time. This was because John Abel, the dean of pharmacologists in this country, purified and crystallized a sample of insulin. When insulin was thus purified, it lost the initial hyperglycemic property.

The early hyperglycemia was attributed to an impurity. Therefore, it was forgotten until 1945, when the notion reappeared through the agency of our old friend, serendipity. A young man by the name of Christian DeDuve, then in Belgium, worked in the laboratory of Bouckaert in Louvain on carbohydrate regulation, using a technique they called normoglycemic compensation. For example, insulin was given to an animal but at the same time glucose was infused through a variable pump to exactly counteract the blood sugar fall. The blood sugar level was kept "normoglycemic." Therefore, the amount of glucose/*kg*/*hr* which was needed to compensate for the hypoglycemic effect of the substance was a measure of insulin action.

Logic would dictate that the more insulin given, the more sugar that would be needed for compensation. DeDuve (1945) found a paradoxical situation when he administered more than seven units of Lilly insulin/*kg*. Less glucose was needed to hold the blood sugar at a normal level than when only six *units*/*kg* were given. At doses of 10 *units*/*kg*, glucose was not needed at all. However, when he used insulin from NOVO the requirement for glucose went up steadily with the dose of insulin. Obviously, the Lilly insulin had in it an "impurity" which was hyperglycemic in effect. The term HGF (hyperglycemic - glycogenolytic factor) was used at first and then the older term glucagon was revived. Glucagon is a peptide produced by a cell that was waiting for the discovery, the cell that Diamare and Lane had written about between 1902 and 1910.

By the early 1950's then, the islets were known to produce two peptide hormones -- insulin in the *beta* cells and glucagon in the *alpha* cells. The more recent developments have consisted of identification of additional cell types and the finding of additional hormonal substances which they elaborate.

By using immunocytochemical techniques as well as electron-microscopy, the following hormonal and neurotransmitter materials have been identified as products of the various cell-types of the islets: (1) insulin, (2) glucagon, (3) somatostatin, (4) pancreatic polypeptide, (5) secretin. In addition, chemical investigations have also shown that the islets contain significant amounts of (a) serotonin and (b) *gamma*-aminobutyric acid (GABA) (Luft and Efendic, 1974; Orci and Amherdt, 1977).

Best known, of course, are the actions of insulin, and this hormone's place in blood-sugar regulation. While much of the pharmacology of glucagon is well established, its precise physiological role and its role in diabetes are still not agreed upon. Somatostatin inhibits the cell secretion of many hormones and enzymes. However, we do not know whether pancreatic somatostatin is ever secreted into the general circulation, or whether it operates by diffusing within the islet system, helping to regulate insulin and/or glucagon secretion. The function of pancreatic polypeptide in man is totally unknown as yet.

In our present state of knowledge, we can ask some intriguing questions, but we will probably have to wait patiently for the answers:

1. How does the set of pancreatic hormones interact with the increasing number of active enteric peptides?
2. Is insulin involved in the maintenance, growth, and secretory activity of the gut epithelium and of the exocrine pancreatic cells?
3. What is the precise relationship of insulin to nerve growth factor, epidermal growth factor, nonspecific insulin-like activity (NSILA), etc.?
4. Is the pituitary growth hormone involved in normal maintenance of islet cells, especially of the β variety?
5. What is the genesis of the β cell hyperplasia in obesity? Does the pancreas produce an insulin-resistance factor?
6. What is the precise physiological interplay in the normal nondiabetic human of glucagon and insulin?

All these and many other legitimate speculations come to mind. The answers, of course, are in the future, but not too far distant. The pace of discovery is now rapid; the wait will be far shorter than the hundred years between Cawley and Minkowski.

REFERENCES

Arnozan, C.L. and Vaillard, L. 1884. Contribution a l'etude de pancreas du lapin. Lesions provoquees par la ligature du canal de Wirsung. *Arch. Physiol. Norm. Path.* 3(3):287-316.

Bensley, R.R. 1911-12. Studies on the pancreas of the guinea pig. *Amer. J. Anat.* 12:297-388.

Bernard, C. 1856. Memoire sur le pancreas. *C.R. Acad. Sci.* Paris, Suppl. 1:379-563.

Bouchardat, A. 1852. Du diabete sucre ou glucosurie. *Mem. Acad. Med.* Paris 16:69-212.

Brisbane, J. 1773. *Select cases in the practice of medicine.* London: G. Scott. (pp 1-11 and 55-62)

Burger, M. and Kramer, H. 1930. Uber die wirkungsverschiedenheit technischer insuline und kristallisirter preparate bezuglich der primaren insulin hyperglykamie. *Arch. Exp. Path. Pharm.* **156**:1.

Cawley, T. 1788. A singular case of diabetes, consisting entirely in the quality of the urine; with an inquiry into the different theories of that disease. *London Med. J.* **9**:286-308.

Chevreul, M.E. 1815. Note sur le sucre de diabete. *Ann. Chim.* Paris **95**:319-320.

DeDuve, C. 1945. *Glucose, insuline et diabete.* Paris: Masson and Cie. (pp XXVII ff and 307)

Diamare, V. 1899. Studii comparativi sulle isole di Langerhans del pancreas. *Intern. Mschr. Anat. Physiol.* **16**:155-209.

Diamare, V. 1924. Documenti per la storia della teoria insulare del diabetes e sui precedenti dell', insulina. *Arch. Fisiol.* Florenz **22**:141-157.

Dieckhoff, C. 1895. Beitrage zur pathologischen anatomie des pankreas mit besonderer berucksichtigung der diabetes-frage. *Beitrage zur Wiss. Med.*:3-146.

Dobson, M. 1776. Experiments and observations on the urine in diabetes. *Med. Obs. Inqui.* **5**:298-316.

Hedon, E. 1892. Greffe sous-cutanee du pancreas: Ses resultats au point de vue de la theorie du diabetes pancreatique. *C.R. Soc. Biol.* Paris **44**:678-680.

Kimball, C.P. and Murlin, J.R. 1923. Aqueous extracts of pancreas. III. Some precipitation reactions of insulin. *J. Biol. Chem.* **58**:337.

Laguesse, E. 1894. Sur la formation des ilots de Langerhans dans le pancreas. *C.R. Soc. Biol.* Paris **46**:819-820.

Laguesse, E. 1910. Importance des ilots endocrines et de leur cycle evolutif dans la physiologie normale et pathologique du pancreas et particulierement dans le diabete. *Presse Med.* **18**:449-453.

Lancereaux, E. 1877. Notes et reflexions a propos de deux cas de diabete sucre avec alteration du pancreas. *Bull. Acad. Med.* Paris **6**:1215-1240.

Lane, W.A. 1907. The cytological characters of the areas of Langerhans. *Amer. J. Anat.* **7**:409-421.

Langerhans, P. 1869. Beitrage zur mikroskopischen anatomie der bauchspeicheldruse. *Med. Diss.* Berlin.

Luft, R., Efendic, S., *et al.* 1974. Immunohistochemical evidence for localization of somatostatin-immunoreactivity in a cell-population of pancreatic-islets. *Med. Biol.* **52**:428.

Mering, J.V. and Minkowski, O. 1889. Diabetes mellitus nach pankreasexstirpation. *Zbl. Klin. Med.* **10**:393-394.

Meyer, J. 1909. Action de la secretion interne du pancreas sur differents organes et en particulier sur la secretion renale. *Arch. Fisiol.* **7**:96-99.

Minkowski, O. 1893. Untersuchungen uber den diabetes mellitus nach exstirpation des pankreas. *Arch. Exp. Path. Pharmak.* 31:85-189.

Minkowski, O. 1929. Die lehre vom pankreas-diabetes in ihrer geschichtlichen entwicklung. *Munch. Med. Wschr.* **76**:311-315.

Orci, L., Amherdt, M., *et al.* 1977. IN Wasiliewski and Chick (Eds.) *Pancreatic beta cell culture.* Amsterdam: Excerpta Medica. (p 9 ff)

Rollo, J. 1797. *An account of two cases of the diabetes mellitus, with remarks as they arose during the progress of the cure.* London: Dilly.

Willis, T. 1674. *Pharmaceutice rationalis* (Chpt. 3). London.

DISCUSSION FOLLOWING DR. LEVINE'S TALK

Question:

May I ask, what is the function of the pancreatic polypeptide as far as you know up to now?

Dr. Levine

I didn't mention it because I really don't know what its function is. I can't find out from anybody else. But it is definitely an entity, it's present in the pancreas, is produced by a specific cell, and can be recognized both by special immunofluorescence and by the shape and size of the granules and the general shape of the cell. But what the physiological function is, is still not known.

Question

Has GABA been localized to the *delta* cell region?

Dr. Levine

No, nobody had yet done immunofluorescence with GABA. Serotonin was, and is, present in those cells where Orci now finds the pancreatic polypeptide. Whether GABA is also present there I have no idea.

Question

Dr. Levine, I wonder if you will comment on the formulation that Dr. Unger published recently in the New England Journal in which he interrelated somatostatin, glucagon, and insulin in controlling the influx and efflux of nutrient fuel into the circulation?

Dr. Levine

Well, I think you will hear here far more authoritatively from Dr. Gerich about those ideas. So I don't want to preempt that discussion now.

Question

Is there not what seems to be a hypothalamic factor for the regulation of these hormones within the pancreas also?

Dr. Levine

The hypothalamus is a small region and almost everything that happens in the central nervous system may eventually have to pass through the midbrain. There are central nervous system effects on the secretion of insulin. They do not seem to be major effects, such as the stimuli by foods and some of the enteric peptides. The parasympathetic nervous system via acetylcholine, seems to have a positive secretory action on *beta* cells. The relation of the central nervous system to the secretion of the other pancreatic hormones is not known.

The sympathetic system inhibits insulin secretion. This is to be expected, since the catecholamines do so.

Question

Dr. Levine, would you care to speculate on what GABA and serotonin do in the islet?

Dr. Levine

No, I have no worthwhile notions about this. When glucagon was found to be an insulin secretagogue it was speculated that it may do by contiguity, since the α and β cells are in close apposition. It may be that serotonin and GABA act "locally" in the way neurohumors do. This is a kind of endocrinology by contact, which is very difficult to explore. Somatostatin presumably may have an influence on both glucagon and insulin secretion within the islet, rather than via the circulation.

Question

Is the GABA transported to the pancreas or is there glutamic decarboxylase in the islets?

Dr. Levine

GABA seems to originate in the pancreas. The decarboxylase is present in amounts similar to those in the central nervous system.

Question

Is the whole GABA cycle there?

Dr. Levine

I don't know whether the whole cycle is present. The decarboxylase definitely is there in high amounts. This was first demonstrated in Japan about two years ago, and has been confirmed.

Question

What is the role of the pancreas in the adult obese diabetes syndrome?

Dr. Levine

In this form of the disease the *beta* cells are not destroyed. The insulin in the blood is high. There is insulin resistance. There is no indication of a possible viral and/or immunological etiology.

It is instructive to consider the diabetes shown by the ob^+/ob^+ mouse. Such animals are obese, hyperglycemic, hyperinsulinemic, and insulin resistant. Severe food restriction brings these signs quickly toward normal. As weight loss goes on, the insulin and the glucose levels fall and sensitivity to insulin is restored.

This is the same regimen which will ameliorate the human adult obese syndrome. In the mouse there is intense islet cell hyperplasia. There are indications that the human syndrome may also exhibit this. The human obese diabetic, when placed on a very low caloric intake (*e.g.*, 400 *cal/day*) will tend to normalize his blood sugar and blood insulin within a period of days, long before there is a significant degree of weight loss. It would seem as if the ordinary traffic of foodstuffs evokes (perhaps via enteric peptides) proliferative activity of the islets, hence increased insulin secretion, lipogenesis, and resistance. Perhaps, then, adult obese diabetes is a disorder stemming either from hyperactivity of gut hormones or from a CNS functional derangement with enhanced appetite and insulin secretion.

Question

Of course, receptors undoubtedly would play a part. How important do you think is the receptor change when insulin action is more adequate, in causing the blood sugar to come down?

Dr. Levine

I do not understand how the slight reduction in the number of measured receptors, let's say 20%-30%, accounts for hyperglycemia. The number of receptors one needs for action seems to be much less than the receptors still present during the insulin-resistant state.

Dr. Hardin

Are there other comments? There are two things that have always amused me about the story of diabetes as it has been so clearly set forth this morning. One is the number of important discoveries that have resulted by accident, serendipity, and the other one which I like to test medical students with, and I hope that there are medical students here today, is the important observations that have been made by students.

We heard this morning about Langerhans finding the islets when he was a senior student. Charley Best contributed to the discovery of insulin when he was a sophomore medical student. These are facts which I relate to students and then ask, "What are you doing this weekend?"

CLINICAL SIGNIFICANCE OF C-PEPTIDE

A.H. Rubenstein and B. Gonen

Department of Medicine
University of Chicago
Chicago, IL 60637

INTRODUCTION

Significant information has accumulated in recent years regarding the biochemical and morphological details of insulin biosynthesis and secretion. Insulin is formed in pancreatic *beta*-cells through enzymatic splitting of a precursor molecule, proinsulin, which itself is a product of the proteolysis of an even larger molecule, preproinsulin (Chan, Keim, and Steiner, 1976; Steiner, 1977; Steiner, Clark, Nolan, Rubenstein, Margoliash, Melani, and Oyer, 1970; Steiner, Kemmler, Clark, Oyer, and Rubenstein, 1972; Steiner and Oyer, 1967). This latter reaction occurs as the molecule traverses the membrane of the rough endoplasmic reticulum. Proinsulin is transported through the cisternal space to the Golgi apparatus, where it is packaged into granules. As the granules mature, proinsulin is cleaved into insulin and C-peptide (Howell, Kostianowski, and Lacy, 1969; Orci, Lambert, Kanazawa, Amherdt, Poviller, and Renold, 1971; Steiner *et al.*, 1972). The molar ratio of C-peptide to insulin equals one in the *beta*-cell granules and portal circulation, but is significantly higher in the peripheral circulation, because of the slower degradation of C-peptide (Horowitz, Starr, Mako, Blackard, and Rubenstein, 1975; Melani, Rubenstein, and Steiner, 1970; Rubenstein, Clark, Melani, and Steiner, 1969).

C-PEPTIDE

Methodology

The establishment of an immunoassay for the determination of circulating C-peptide has encountered some difficulties, because of the poor immunogenicity of C-peptide and the necessity to use synthetic C-peptide as a standard. In addition, circulating C-peptide is heterogeneous, with various closely related peptides having different immunogenic properties.

Because the C-peptide sequence is contained within the proinsulin molecule, antisera prepared against C-peptide also react with proinsulin. The contribution of serum proinsulin to total serum C-peptide immunoreactivity (CPR) is usually small (less than 3%), because of its low concentration in serum. In conditions where the proinsulin levels are elevated, the contribution of proinsulin to total C-peptide immunoreactivity increases markedly. In order to measure C-peptide specifically, proinsulin can be removed from serum by binding to anti-insulin antibodies coupled to Sepharose beads. As mentioned previously, binding of proinsulin to circulating anti-insulin antibodies in the plasma of insulin-treated diabetic patients prolongs its half-life and increases its contribution to C-peptide immunoreactivity. A preliminary step involving precipitation of insulin antibodies (*e.g.*, with the use of polyethylene glycol) removes the bound proinsulin and, thus, enables the direct estimation of the free C-peptide in the supernatant.

C-peptide Levels in Juvenile Onset Diabetes

Insulin deficiency is the basic underlying defect in patients with Type I diabetes mellitus. However, estimation of circulating insulin levels is difficult once exogenous insulin therapy has been initiated. Measurement of endogenously secreted insulin became possible following the development of an immunoassay for circulating C-peptide (Block, Mako, and Steiner, 1972; Heding, 1978; Melani *et al.*, 1970). Quantitation of serum C-peptide has provided the means to gain insight into the natural course of *beta*-cell function, as well as into the effect of residual *beta*-cell function on metabolic control, in Type I diabetic patients. The following discussion will concentrate mainly on the contribution that C-peptide measurements have made to our understanding of various aspects of insulin-dependent diabetes mellitus.

During episodes of ketoacidosis C-peptide was undetectable in patients' sera (Block *et al.*, 1972). Clinical remission, characterized by improved metabolic control and decrease in insulin requirements, was associated with partial functional recovery of *beta*-cell secretory ability as assessed by serum C-peptide determinations. The clinical remission typically occurs in insulin-requiring juvenile onset diabetic patients within a few weeks, or months, following the diagnosis of the diabetic state (Faber and Binder, 1977a; Ludvigsson and Heding, 1978).

The recent development of a more sensitive method for assaying C-peptide has facilitated the undertaking of more detailed studies regarding the time course of the deterioration in *beta*-cell secretory capacity. Ludvigsson and Heding (1978) followed 12 diabetic children from the time of diagnosis for approximately one year with frequent serum C-peptide measurements. At the time of diagnosis all patients had very low, but measurable, C-peptide levels. After approximately one month all patients entered a period of clinical remission, during which an increase in fasting C-peptide concentrations was noted. Over the following nine months there was a steady decrease in serum C-peptide levels, with values in the normal range in only one of eight patients. When a group of 93 insulin-requiring children, diabetic for longer than two years, was studied (Ludvigsson and Heding, 1978), 35% had detectable fasting serum C-peptide levels (>0.04 *pmol/ml*). Of these 34 children, 19 had levels below, 12 had levels within, and three had levels above the range found in normal children.

In an investigation of 35 diabetic patients with a mean duration of diabetes of 4.8 years, 71% had detectable C-peptide levels in their serum (Grajwer, Pildes, Horwitz, and Rubenstein, 1977). Another study (Hendriksen, Faber, Drejer, and Binder, 1977) has shown C-peptide levels >0.03 *pmol/ml* in 76% of diabetic patients with an average duration of insulin therapy of 12 years. Finally, Faber and Binder (1977a) studied 17 insulin-requiring diabetic patients within two to four weeks of initiation of insulin therapy. All patients has measurable C-peptide levels, ranging from 0.08 - 0.45 *pmol/ml* (mean value: 0.17 *pmol/ml*; mean value for healthy controls: 0.36 *pmol/ml*). Following the ingestion of a meal there was a significant rise in serum C-peptide levels in the diabetic patients, but its magnitude was smaller and its appearance delayed when compared to the response in the controls. It can be concluded from these studies that: (a) the deterioration of *beta* cell function, which occurs almost invariably in insulin-requiring diabetic patients, may have a protracted course over many years. Whether the final destruction is the result of an ongoing process in the pancreas or a consequence of repeated insults cannot be answered at present. (b) Periods of clinical remission are associated with partial recovery of insulin secretion by the *beta* cells.

Assessment of pancreatic insulin reserve was also carried out by measuring C-peptide in the stimulated state after either an intravenous injection of 1 *mg* glucagon or the ingestion of a meal. Faber and Binder (1977b) found an increase in C-peptide levels in response to each of these stimuli in 90% of insulin-dependent diabetic patients, whose disease had lasted less than two years at the time of the study. There was a significant correlation between the magnitude of the C-peptide response and the basal C-peptide values. When patients with longer duration of diabetes

(Hendriksen *et al.*, 1977) were subjected to the same two stimuli, the prevalence of preserved, though reduced, *beta* cell function fell to 43% (36 out of 83 patients), with the highest insulinogenic reserve being present in the patients with the shortest duration of diabetes. None of the patients with undetectable fasting C-peptide responded to glucagon stimulation with a rise in C-peptide concentration, whereas all 29 patients with fasting C-peptide greater than 0.08 *pmol/ml* had a significant response to the test. In a report by Ludvigsson and Heding (1977), the glucagon test was performed in 10 insulin-requiring diabetic children, and only three had a slight increase in their C-peptide levels. The rise in C-peptide following either stimulation test (glucagon or meal) was similar, permitting these tests to be used interchangeably. Thus, the use of a simple and rapid test (*i.e.*, glucagon injection) can help assess the physiological response of endogenous *beta*-cell-secretory function.

C-PEPTIDE AND METABOLIC CONTROL

As pointed out, there is evidence that the period of clinical remission in juvenile onset diabetic patients is, at least partially, due to the recovery of the insulin secretory capacity of the *beta* cells. The patients with the highest serum C-peptide concentrations had the lowest requirement for exogenous insulin (Faber and Binder, 1977a) and also had the most stable metabolic status (as defined by blood glucose excursions around meals). There is, as yet, little information pertaining to the quantitative aspect of *beta* cell reserve, although Hendriksen *et al.* (1977) have concluded that a serum C-peptide level of 0.07 *pmol/ml* or greater should be considered significant.

The influence of persistent C-peptide secretion on diabetic control and stability at times unrelated to the remission period has been the subject of a number of studies. Shima, Tanaka, Morishita, Tarui, Kumahara, and Nishikawa (1977) measured fasting C-peptide levels in 46 insulin-requiring diabetic patients, in whom diabetic instability was assessed by the sum of standard deviations of 10 fasting glucose levels taken on different days. The results showed that the patients with the highest C-peptide values had the most stable diabetes. Similar results were reported by Grajwer *et al.* (1977); Reynolds, Molnar, Horwitz, Rubenstein, Taylor, and Tiang (1977); Yue, Baxter, and Turtle (1977). Finally, we have recently demonstrated, using hemoglobin A1 measurement as an indicator of metabolic control, that in nonobese insulin-treated subjects fasting C-peptide levels correlated significantly with the degree of diabetic control.

ACKNOWLEDGMENTS

Supported by grants from the Bertha and Henry Brownstein Foundation, Chicago and the National Institutes of Health AM 13941 and AM 20595.

REFERENCES

Block, M.B., Mako, M.E., Steiner, D.F., and Rubenstein, A.H. 1972. Curculating C-peptide immunoreactivity: Studies in normals and diabetic patients. *Diabetes* **21**:1013-1026.

Chan, S.J., Keim, P., and Steiner, D.F. 1976. Cell free synthesis of rat preproinsulins: Characterization and partial amino acid sequence determination. *Proc. Nat'l. Acad. Sci.* USA **73**:1964-1968.

Faber, O.K. and Binder, C. 1977a. β-cell function and blood glucose control in insulin dependent diabetes within the first month of insulin treatment. *Diabetologia* **13**:263-268.

Faber, O.K. and Binder, C. 1977b. C-peptide response to glucagon. A test for the residual *beta* cell function in diabetes mellitus. *Diabetes* **26**:605-610.

Grajwer, L.A., Pildes, R.S., Horwitz, D.L., and Rubenstein, A.H. 1977. Control of juvenile diabetes mellitus and its relationship to endogenous insulin secretion as measured by C-peptide immunoreactivity. *J. Pediat.* **90**:42-48.

Heding, L.G. 1978. Insulin, C-peptide and proinsulin in non diabetics and insulin treated diabetics. *Diabetes* **27**:178-183. (Suppl. 1)

Hendriksen, C., Faber, O.K., Drejer, T., and Binder, C. 1977. Prevalence of residual *beta* cell function in insulin treated diabetics evaluated on the C-peptide response to intravenous glucagon. *Diabetologia* **13**:280-288.

Horwitz, D.L., Starr, J.I., Mako, M.E., Blackard, W.G., and Rubenstein, A.H. 1975. Proinsulin, insulin, and C-peptide concentrations in human portal and peripheral blood. *J. Clin. Invest.* **55**:1278-1283.

Howell, S.L., Kostianowski, M., and Lacy, P.E. 1969. *Beta* granule formation in isolated islets of Langerhans: A study by electron microscopic radioautography. *J. Cell Biol.* **42**:695-705.

Ludvigsson, J. and Heding, L.G. 1977. C-peptide in diabetic children after stimulation with glucagon compared with fasting C-peptide levels in non-diabetic children. *Acta Endocrinol.* **85**:364-371.

Ludvigsson, J. and Heding, L.G. 1978. *Beta* cell function in children with diabetes. *Diabetes* **27**:230-234. (Suppl. 1)

Melani, F., Rubenstein, A.H., Oyer, P.E., and Steiner, D.F. 1970. Identification of proinsulin and C-peptide in human serum by a specific immunoassay. *Proc. Nat'l. Acad. Sci.* USA **67**:148-155.

Orci, L., Lambert, A.E., Kanazawa, Y., Amherdt, M., Poviller, C., and Renold, A.E. 1971. Morphologic and biochemical studies of β cells of fetal rat endocrine pancreas in organ culture. Evidence for proinsulin biosynthesis. *J. Cell Biol.* **50**:565-582.

Reynolds, C., Molnar, G.D., Horwitz, D.L., Rubenstein, A.H., Taylor, W.F., and Tiang, N-S. 1977. Abnormalities of endogenous glucagon and insulin in unstable diabetes. *Diabetes* **26**:36-45.

Rubenstein, A.H., Clark, J.L., Melani, F., and Steiner, D.F. 1969. Secretion of proinsulin C-peptide by pancreatic *beta* cells and its circulation in blood. *Nature* **224**:697-699.

Shima, K., Tanaka, R., Morishita, S., Tarui, S., Kumahara, Y., and Nishikawa, M. 1977. Studies on the etiology of brittle diabetes. Relationship between diabetic instability and insulinogenic reserve. *Diabetes* **26**:717-725.

Steiner, D.F. 1977. Insulin today. *Diabetes* **26**:322-340.

Steiner, D.F., Clark, J.L., Nolan, C., Rubenstein, A.H., Margoliash, E., Melani, F., and Oyer, P.E. 1970. The biosynthesis of insulin and some speculations regarding the pathogenesis of human diabetes. pp. 57-80. **IN** E. Cerasi and R. Luft (Eds.) *Novel symposium thirteen on pathogenesis of diabetes mellitus.* Stockholm: Almquist and Wiksell.

Steiner, D.F., Kemmler, W., Clark, J.L., Oyer, P.E., and Rubenstein, A.H. 1972. The biosynthesis of insulin. pp. 175-193. **IN** D.F. Steiner and N. Freinkel (Eds.) *Handbook of physiology.* Section 7: Endocrinology 1, *Endocrine pancreas.* Washington, DC: Amer. Physiol. Soc.

Steiner, D.F. and Oyer, P.E. 1967. The biosynthesis of insulin and a probable precursor of insulin by a human islet cell adenoma. *Proc. Nat'l. Acad. Sci.* USA **57**:473-480.

Yue, D.K., Baxter, R.C., and Turtle, J.R. 1977. C-peptide secretion and insulin antibodies as determinants of stability in diabetes mellitus. *Metabolism* **27**:35-41.

DISCUSSION FOLLOWING DR. RUBENSTEIN'S TALK

Dr. Sperling

I'm fascinated by the values which you have recorded from some of the diabetics with measurable C-peptide. In some of your earlier slides you indicated that the C-peptide level normally was of the order of one to two *ng/mℓ* and rose to a value of approximately five *ng/mℓ* during stimulation with oral glucose. Yet, in one of the later slides, you pointed out that the diabetics who are easy to control segregated with C-peptide values that were as high as seven *ng/mℓ* in the basal state, which is somewhere of the order of three to five times as high as normal. I wonder whether this is all C-peptide or whether an equally adequate explanation might be that there are antibodies directed against insulin as a result of insulin therapy, that these antibodies to insulin bind proinsulin and prevent its degradation, and this bound proinsulin is reacting in the C-peptide radioimmunoassay. Could the reason for these patients showing good stability be that they have these antibodies which bind insulin and release it on a prolonged basis as the need arises, rather than that the patients have C-peptide or residual insulin secretory ability?

Dr. Rubenstein

Yes, the explanation of the high values is just as you have said. We've pointed this out many times. I didn't really want to belabor the point today in an overview. Many of these patients have insulin antibodies and we've found that these insulin antibodies bind not only insulin but proinsulin via its insulin moiety. The proinsulin, which is secreted in relatively small amounts, then accumulates in the bloodstream bound to these antibodies which have a very slow turnover, a half-life of maybe 18 days or so. The antibodies to C-peptide that we use in the immunoassay do cross react with the C-peptide part of proinsulin as well as with the free C-peptide. Many of those values of "total C-peptide" do indicate *beta* cell function on a qualitative basis but, as you have pointed out, on a quantitative basis the values have to be interpreted with caution.

We've now published (Kuzuya *et al.*, 1977) rather simple techniques to separate the proinsulin bound onto antibodies from the free

C-peptide. With polyethylene glycol, which precipitates large proteins, one can precipitate the antibodies with insulin and proinsulin attached, and then measure the C-peptide free in the supernate. Using this rather simple approach one can obtain quantitative values for free C-peptide in diabetic patients who have insulin antibodies.

I don't agree with the second point you made. There has been a lot of discussion in the literature as to whether one can equate diabetic control with the possibility that the antibodies are important because they bind insulin and delay insulin action. Nevertheless, there have been some rather good studies which point out that antibodies probably contribute little in terms of affecting diabetic control. In fact, in Europe there are large numbers of diabetic patients now being treated with monocomponent insulin who do not even, after a couple of years, have a significant titer of insulin antibodies. Interestingly, those patients are no different in terms of their ability to be controlled than patients who have an appreciable level of antibodies. Of course, there are some patients who have a very high titer of antibodies and they may have insulin resistance due to the antibodies. There also are a small number of patients who have antibodies with low capacity and high affinity. Dixon *et al.* (1972), and I think we agree, have suggested that these patients may be very "brittle" because of the unusual character of their antibodies. In general, I think that antibodies play a rather minor role in terms of diabetic control while the absorption and degradation of insulin from the tissue site where it is injected is probably the major factor.

Dr. Werner

Drs. Gerich and Forsham have shown a "blunting" effect of the *alpha* cell response to hypoglycemia in juvenile onset diabetes. Many of these patients are unstable diabetics, like this group that you have studied. Is there any correlation between the ones who do have blunted response to hypoglycemia and those who still have C-reactive peptide?

Dr. Rubenstein

That is something that intrigued us a great deal: that is, whether the loss in *alpha* cell recognition of glucose or response to hypoglycemia, as Gerich *et al.* (1973) pointed out, could be correlated with the degree of loss of *beta* cell function. Reynolds *et al.* (1977) studied that question and were able to show a rather good correlation between the loss of ability of *alpha* cells to respond to hypoglycemia with glucagon output and the C-peptide stimulatibility of the *beta* cells. In fact, there is a study from Japan which looked at this question from another point-of-view and came to the same conclusion: that the degree of loss of *beta* cell function correlates rather well with the degree of loss of *alpha* cell function in terms of glucose recognition (Shima *et al.*, 1977).

On the other hand, these *alpha* cells respond well to arginine and may even hyperrespond. It thus seems that they are not glucagon-deficient in the way that the *beta* cells are insulin-deficient, but have lost the ability to monitor, or recognize, glucose, or they may need insulin to recognize changes in glucose levels efficiently. One of the implications might be -- that the hypoglycemic attacks, which are another feature of difficult control, in these patients, may be aggravated by the fact that they can't put out glucagon in response to the hypoglycemia. So the defect, as Unger pointed out, in terms of their ability to maintain a stable blood sugar level may be affected in two ways. Not only do they not have enough insulin to keep their blood sugar normal but, when you try to normalize their glucose with exogenous insulin and overshoot slightly, their ability to respond with glucagon output is impaired. As Molnar pointed out in 1974, many of these patients have wide swings in their blood sugar concentrations as part of their poor control.

Dr. Park

I would like to ask you about your "pre-pro" story. Have those "pre"-peptides been analyzed now and is the nature of how they bind to the membrane understood? And are they all hydrophobic residues? Is there any similarity among the various "pre's?"

Dr. Rubenstein

There have been partial sequences of about four or five of these peptides. They do have small regions of homology which, as you point out, may be strongly hydrophobic. So although they have regions which are heterologous, there does seem to be some conservation of structure.

Dr. Steffes

Are the C-peptide levels routinely elevated in the well controlled as compared to poorly controlled diabetic patients? Are they elevated at all times or just after meals? If they are consistently at a higher level and yet provide better control, it may be important in evaluating other modalities of treating diabetes.

Dr. Rubenstein

I think that the best study along those lines is one by Faber and Binder (1977). They studied patients who were euglycemic and then induced mild hypoglycemia and thereafter gave them a meal. They studied whether their residual *beta* secretory ability responded similarly to normals. In fact, they did. When these patients are hyperglycemic, they secrete as much C-peptide (insulin) as they can, which is perhaps a third, or a quarter, or a tenth of normal. If you make them hypoglycemic they suppress their C-peptide output.

Thus, it appears that those cells which are left have normal control mechanisms. When we see a steady level, it's because they are hyperglycemic and secreting maximally. If you normalize their blood sugar with insulin they respond like normals, but at a lower level.

I also pointed out, at least in a very preliminary sense, something that Dr. Jackson has implied very often. If you can normalize the blood sugar of these patients for several days and then give them a *beta* cell secretagogue, they secrete more insulin than if you test them at a time when they have been hyperglycemic. Thus hyperstimulation of the *beta* cell may exhaust its secretory reserve.

Dr. Levine

What is the behavior of the C-peptide in the fasting state and after standard meals in the heterogenous group of the so-called adult onset diabetics, especially those with obesity? Does it give any indication that you can follow the dynamics of synthesis?

Dr. Rubenstein

Essentially, what it shows is that the values are as predictable as those of insulin. It really gave us no better information.

Dr. Levine

Than the insulin itself?

Dr. Rubenstein

We might have hoped there would be a discrepancy between insulin and C-peptide or that the liver would take up more, or less, insulin in these patients. However, the data have not turned out like that. The correlation between insulin and C-peptide in normals and in maturity onset diabetics is similar. So we haven't found any surprises in that group of patients by measuring C-peptide.

Dr. Burns

I was a little concerned about the timetable of deterioration of the C-peptide levels in new diabetics. As I recall your one slide, it decreased by half in 12 months, and then you said approached zero at three or four years.

I think all of us who take care of diabetics see individuals who go for years with requirements of 20 to 25 units daily, either in two doses or one, which would suggest that they are retaining *beta* cell function. I wonder if you have had an opportunity to see if this is verified or confirmed by C-peptide measurements?

Dr. Rubenstein

Yes. The group I showed were children. When we studied adults the pattern was different. If one studies insulin-requiring adult onset patients, beginning at the age of 20, 30, or 40, it is interesting because most of them are very different from children. A minority look like the children, but the majority lose less *beta* cell function and retain this secretory capacity for long periods of time. These are the patients who often manage well taking one injection of insulin per day. They can exercise or miss a meal and seldom have problems. We can predict from their clinical course that these patients will have appreciable amounts of C-peptide in their plasma, and they do. The severe loss is confined to young patients, and a minority of older patients.

Dr. Jackson

Just a brief comment regarding the degree and duration of partial remission in children after the onset of overt insulin-dependend diabetes. In our experience the maintenance exogenous insulin requirement per unit of body weight varies depending on how early the diagnosis is made and how soon adequate insulin treatment is given. The earlier the diagnosis was made, the lower the amount of insulin needed and the easier it was to attain and maintain a high degree of control with little risk of even a mild insulin reaction. The maintenance insulin requirement for children with early diagnosis and treatment may be as low as 0.10 to 0.25 *units/kg/day*, and the period of partial remission may persist for a period of years; whereas, the insulin requirement for children with delayed treatment usually exceeds 0.50 *units/kg/day*, and their period of partial remission invariably persists for only a few months.

Recently we have documented by C-peptide measurements that children with overt diabetes who are maintained in metabolic control are producing variable amounts of endogenous insulin. We have found a close correlation between the children's maintenance exogenous insulin requirement per unit of ideal body weight and their postprandial C-peptide level after the ingestion of a standardized liquid meal. Children requiring over 0.65 *units/kg/day* no longer have a detectable postprandial C-peptide serum level.

On the basis of serial oral glucose tolerance tests done on siblings of children with overt diabetes, we have observed a number of children with borderline, or definitely abnormal tests, during their prepubescent growth spurts, which have reverted to normal after maturation and cessation of their linear growth. We also have observed a few postpubescent girls with recent onset of overt insulin-dependent diabetes who have had a very low insulin requirement and a more prolonged period of partial remission. Consequently, it is not surprising that young adults with recent onset of overt diabetes may continue to produce varying amounts of endogenous insulin for prolonged periods of time.

Dr. Clements

What decides the time course of proinsulin-insulin conversion? What evidence do you have that the proinsulin-converting enzymes are actually localized to the bilayer of the insulin granule membrane rather than to the matrix?

Dr. Rubenstein

The studies of Kemmler and Steiner (1970) have shown that converting ability is retained in the membrane fraction of the isolated granules. The quantity of enzymes in the granules is extremely low and this has made it very difficult to purify them.

Dr. Bar

If a child develops diabetes, goes through a transition period of having some C-peptide activity, and later in his course has no measurable C-peptide, is that *beta* cell function irretrievably lost?

Dr. Rubenstein

Well, there will be some time when *beta* cell function will be completely lost and there will be an earlier time when there will be residual secretory capacity.

What I'm saying is that if the children are hyperglycemic, then you may exhaust their *beta* cell reserve at a time when some *beta* cells are still alive. Therefore, if you render them euglycemic, they will probably synthesize small amounts of insulin and have a small amount of residual secretory capacity. Further on in their course you can make them euglycemic and *beta* cell function will not recover. I must say that we have been impressed that even a small amount of *beta* cell secretory capacity may be important.

Dr. Shear

I gather that the C-peptide has no biologic activity itself and no feedback control on endocrine glands, is that the case?

Dr. Rubenstein

We have looked very hard but without success to find a new function for the C-peptide. We had a number of wonderful ideas, *e.g.*, that it was the peptide that regulated the satiety site in the brain.

It still seems to me that there should be a function, but this now seems unlikely. Steiner suggests that its function is to permit α and β chain apposition and after that it is just disposed of through the plasma. But I have a prejudice that we'll find something.

Dr. Heimberg

You talked about abnormal amino acid sequences in your proinsulin. Have you ever seen any abnormal sequences not only in the proinsulin molecules but in the insulin molecules?

Dr. Rubenstein

Well, we haven't got that far yet, but we are studying some patients who we believe might have this problem. These patients have very high insulin levels and yet they are hyperglycemic. They do not seem to have any receptor problem and they respond to exogenous insulin normally. So the kind of simple explanation is that they have a lot of insulin but it is not working. Our preliminary data tend to indicate that we may be dealing with an abnormal insulin. It is an insulin which has low biological activity compared to control insulin purified from a normal person's plasma. We have a long way to go to show that, but we're excited by the possibility that we may have the tools now to identify not only defects in the conversion, but in the actual insulin molecule itself.

Question

Do you find any kind of relation between the C-peptide and glucagon?

Dr. Rubenstein

No. The C-peptide normally correlates with insulin, but just as insulin doesn't correlate with glucagon, so the C-peptide seems to be independent.

DISCUSSION REFERENCES

Dixon, K., Exon, P.D., and Hughes, H.R. 1972. Insulin antibodies in aetiology of labile diabetes. *Lancet* **1**:343-347.

Faber, O.K. and Binder, C. 1977. β-cell function and blood glucose control in insulin dependent diabetics within the first month of insulin treatment. *Diabetologia* **13**:263-268.

Kemmler, W. and Steiner, D.F. 1970. Conversion of proinsulin to insulin in a subcellular fraction from rat islets. *Biochem. Biophys. Res. Comm.* **41**:1223-1230.

Kuzuya, H., Blix, P.M., Horwitz, D.L., Steiner, D.F., and Rubenstein, A.H. 1977. Determination of free and total insulin and C-peptide in insulin-treated diabetics. *Diabetes* **26**:22-29.

Molnar, G.D., Taylor, W.F., and Langworthy, A. 1974. On measuring the adequacy of diabetes regulation: Comparison of continuously monitored blood glucose patterns with values at selected time points. *Diabetologia* **10**:139-143.

Reynolds, C., Molnar, G.D., Horwitz, D.L., Rubenstein, A.H., Taylor, W.F., and Jiang, N-S. 1977. Abnormalities of endogenous glu-

cagon and insulin in unstable diabetics. *Diabetes* **26**:36-45.
Shima, K., Tanaka, R., Morishita, S., Tarui, S., Kumahara, Y., and Nishikawa, M. 1977. Studies on the etiology of "brittle" diabetes. Relationship between diabetic instability and insulinogenic reserve. *Diabetes* **26**:717-725.

GLUCAGON: SECRETION AND ACTIONS

Mark A. Sperling[1]

Children's Hospital Medical Center
Elland and Bethesda Avenues
Cincinnati, OH 45229

OUTLINE

Introduction

- Heterogeneity of Circulating Glucagon
- Sources of Circulating Glucagon

Control of Glucagon Secretion

- Nutrients
- Autonomic Influences on Glucagon Secretion
- Parasympathetic
- Miscellaneous Factors Affecting Glucagon Secretion

Glucagon Action

Glucagon in the Newborn Period

Significance of Glucagon Secretion and Action

INTRODUCTION

The role of glucagon in normal glucose homeostasis and the potential contribution of this hormone to the genesis and maintenance of the hyperglycemia and ketonemia of diabetes mellitus have been the focus of extensive investigation in the past decade. Re-

---

[1]Original research of the author supported, in part, by USPHS Grant HD-07087 from the NICHD of NIH, Bethesda, MD, and by the Juvenile Diabetes Foundation. Dr. Sperling is a recipient of a Research Career Development Award from the United State Public Health Service (1 KO 4 HD-00029).

cent studies have affirmed the participation and importance of glucagon in the control of hepatic glucose output (Bomboy, Jr., Lewis, Sinclair-Smith, Lacy, and Liljenquist, 1977a; Bomboy, Lewis, Lacy, Sinclair-Smith, and Liljenquist, 1977b; Chiasson, Liljenquist, Jennings, Keller, and Lacy, 1976; Felig, Wahren, and Hendler, 1976a), but at the same time challenged its significance for the genesis of the metabolic abnormalities of diabetes (Felig *et al.*, 1976b). Two major tools have enabled the performance of these studies. The first is the availability of radioimmunoassay procedures utilizing antisera with a high degree of "specificity" for so-called pancreatic glucagon (Sperling, DeLamater, Kazenelson, Fiser, and Fisher, 1974). The second is the availability of somatostatin (SRIF), the tetradecapeptide which inhibits the secretion of a number of hormones including insulin and glucagon (Vale, Brazeau, Rivier, Brown, Boss, Rivier, Burgus, Ling, and Guillemin, 1975). Thus, it has proved possible to define plasma glucagon concentrations under a variety of normal, or abnormal, circumstances and to define glucagon's contribution through selective administration of this hormone, insulin, or both, at doses designed to achieve the desired plasma concentration during ongoing SRIF infusion. This review will focus on current understanding of the factors controlling the secretion of glucagon and its contribution to the control of metabolism in health and disease.

Heterogeneity of Circulating Glucagon

A major problem in the interpretation of results has been the wide discrepancy in basal plasma glucagon concentrations reported by different authors using different specific antisera; basal values have ranged from a low of 18 *pg/ml* (Alford, Bloom, and Nabarro, 1977; Matsuyama, Hoffman, Dunbar, Foa, and Foa, 1976) to as high as 275 *pg/ml* (Kuku, Zeidler, Emmanouel, Katz, and Rubenstein, 1976). Even with the same antiserum, reported basal values in separate laboratories have differed by as much as 100 *pg/ml*, and as much as 50 *pg/ml* in the same laboratory in separate studies. These discrepancies and inconsistencies have relevance for the dispute in studies which report the presence, or absence, of measurable glucagon in pancreatectomized man (Barnes and Bloom, 1976) and, consequently, the significance of glucagon in the genesis of diabetic ketoacidosis (Barnes, Bloom, Alberti, Smythe, Alford, and Chisholm, 1977). Most investigators now report basal values in the range of 50 to 150 *pg/ml* and, although quantitatively different, studies of the factors which stimulate or suppress plasma glucagon concentrations are qualitatively similar.

Not all of the measured plasma glucagon represents the biologically most potent form of the hormone, which contains 29 amino acids and has a molecular weight of 3500 *daltons*. Elution profiles after gel chromatography of plasma reveal a large fraction of measured glucagon eluting with the void volume corresponding to a molecular weight equal to or greater than γ globulin, an intermediate form corresponding to a *MW* of approximately 9000, as well as the 3500 *MW* form, which may account for only 10% to 60% of total measured glucagon (Kuku *et al.*, 1976). The proportion of this smaller form is raised in ketoacidosis (Kuku *et al.*, 1976) as well as in patients with glucagon-secreting tumors (Boden and Owen, 1977). In patients with renal failure, total plasma glucagon is elevated and gel chromatography reveals the largest fraction in the intermediate 9000 *MW* form (Kuku *et al.*, 1976). That this material is less biologically active is suggested from studies in a family with hyperglucagonemia but without evidence of disturbed carbohydrate metabolism (Boden and Owen, 1977); such individuals may provide clues for abnormalities in the synthetic sequence of glucagon analogous to the recently described familial abnormality in insulin synthesis (Gabbay, DeLuca, Fisher, Mako, and Rubenstein, 1976). Other elegant studies have convincingly demonstrated that the large molecular forms of glucagon are less active biologically (Sasaki, Rubalcava, Baetens, Blazques, Srikant, Orci, and Unger, 1975).

Sources of Circulating Glucagon

The major source of glucagon secretion is the α-cells of the islets of Langerhans. Cells indistinguishable by electron microscopy, and secreting a material which is identical by chemical, immunological and biological criteria to pancreatic glucagon, are found in the gastrointestinal tract (Sasaki *et al.*, 1975). These cells have been well characterized in the gastric fundus of the dog but not well characterized in man (Sasaki *et al.*, 1975; Srikant, McCorkle, and Unger, 1977). In addition, there are scattered throughout the gastrointestinal tract, including in the salivary glands, cells which resemble pancreatic α-cells but which are clearly distinguishable (Lawrence, Tan, Hojvat, and Kirsteins, 1977; Sasaki *et al.*, 1975; Srikant *et al.*, 1977). These cells produce a material(s) which cross reacts to some extent with antisera to glucagon and, consequently, has been termed glucagon-like immunoreactivity (GLI) or "gut" glucagon (Lawrence *et al.*, 1977; Sasaki *et al.*, 1975; Srikant *et al.*, 1977; Valverde, Dobbs, and Unger, 1975). One form of gut glucagon has recently been characterized. It has been termed "glycentin" because it contains 100 amino acid residues; within the last 36 or so amino acids may be contained the entire 29 amino acid sequence of pancreatic glucagon (Sundby, Jacobsen, and Moodly, 1976). Thus, cross reactivity with glucagon antisera is not surprising, although the biological significance of these materials remains enigmatic.

CONTROL OF GLUCAGON SECRETION

The control of glucagon secretion is accomplished through the integrated action of nutrients, in concert with the autonomic nervous system and the prevailing milieu of hormones and ions (Unger, 1974; Woods and Porte, 1974).

Nutrients

Glucose exerts a profound modulating effect on glucagon secretion under normal circumstances (Unger, 1974). A rapid fall in pancreatic glucagon secretion occurs when glucose is raised from 100 mg/dℓ to 150 mg/dℓ (Figure 1). In the isolated perfused pancreas, no further fall in glucagon secretion occurs when glucose concentration is raised above 150 mg/dℓ. The extraordinary sensitivity of this response is evident when step increase, or decreases, from normal glucose concentration are introduced. The fall in glucagon is greatest with the initial 10 mg/dℓ increment in glucose; subsequent increments produce successively less fall (Figure 2).

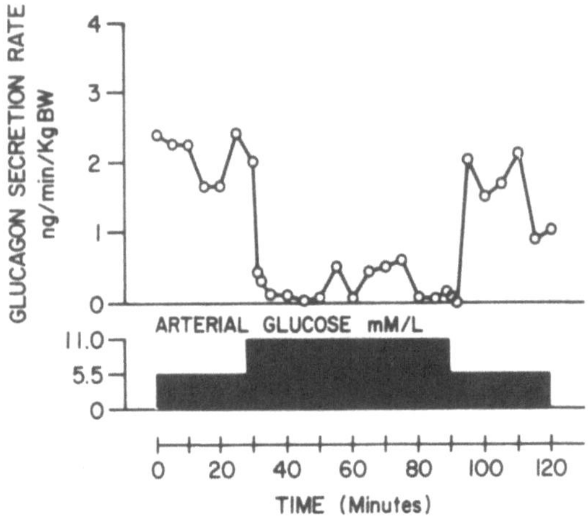

Figure 1. The effect of glucose on glucagon secretion rate (GSR) in the isolated blood-perfused canine pancreas. Note the rapidity with which GSR falls to near zero levels when the glucose concentration is raised from 5.5 mM to 11.0 mM (100-200 mg/dℓ) and the rapid restoration of GSR when glucose is lowered.

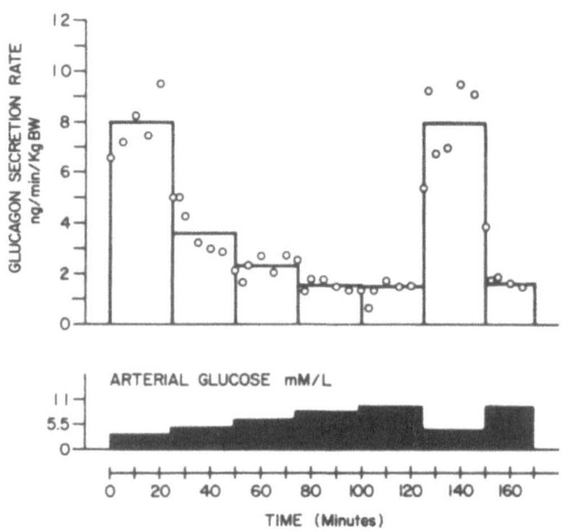

Figure 2. The effect of step increases of 1.1 mM (20 mg/dℓ) in glucose concentration on glucagon secretion rate (GSR) in the isolated blood-perfused canine pancreas. Note the sensitivity to the initial increment of glucose and progressively smaller sensitivity thereafter. No further fall in GSR occurs above glucose concentrations of 8.8 mM (approximately 150 mg/dℓ).

Conversely, the greatest rise in glucagon occurs when glucose is approaching basal concentration after an initial high level (Figure 3). Similarly, in man glucagon falls after glucose ingestion (Figure 4), the magnitude of the fall being approximately 30% to

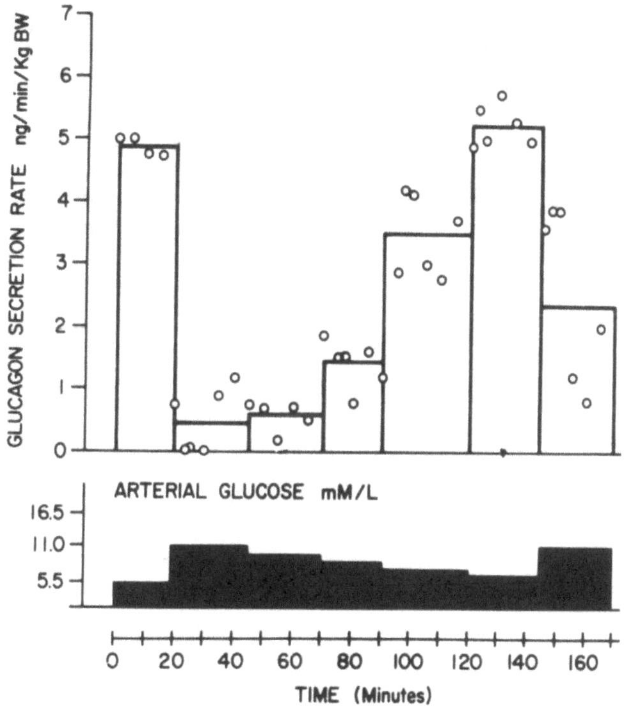

Figure 3. The effect of step increases of 1.1 mM (20 mg/dℓ) in glucose concentration on glucagon secretion rate (GSR) in the isolated blood-perfused canine pancreas. Note the progressively greater response in GSR as glucose approaches 5.5 mM (100 mg/dℓ), and the smaller increments in GSR at higher glucose concentrations.

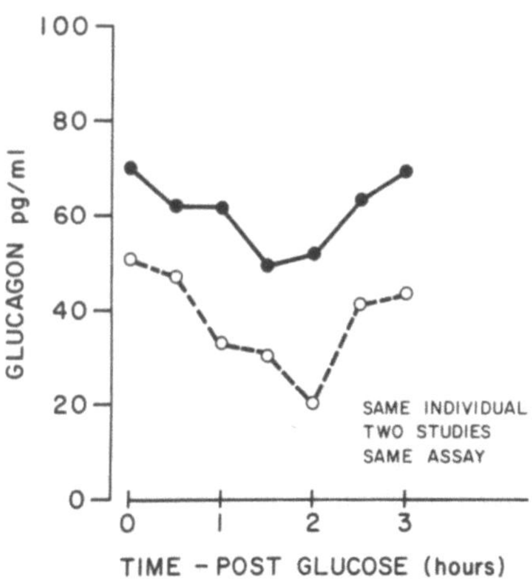

Figure 4. Glucagon response during oral glucose tolerance tests in man. Note the variability in response of the same individual studied on two separate occasions. The suppression of glucagon is consistent and of the order of 30% - 50% from basal.

50% from basal, while glucagon rises when glucose falls as a result of fasting (Aguilar-Parada, Eisentraut, and Unger, 1969), reactive hypoglycemia (Gerich, Schneider, Dippe, Langlois, Noacco, Karam, and Forsham, 1974), and with insulin (Gerich *et al.*, 1974) or ethanol-induced hypoglycemia (Palmer and Ensinck, 1975). Numerous studies suggest that the glucose-induced fall in glucagon is dependent on the availability of insulin (Bratten, Faloona, and Unger, 1974; Gerich, Tsalikian, Lorenzi, Schneider, Bohannon, Gustafson, and Karam, 1975d; Muller, Faloona, and Unger, 1971a: Raskin, Fujita, and Unger, 1975; Sperling, Aleck, and Voina, 1977b; Unger, Aguilar-Parada, Muller, and Eisentraut, 1970). Thus, there is no fall in glucagon despite existent and/or induced hyperglycemia in insulin-dependent diabetics, but a normal response can be restored with concomitant insulin administration or after a period of strict control (Figure 5). Indeed, a relation between

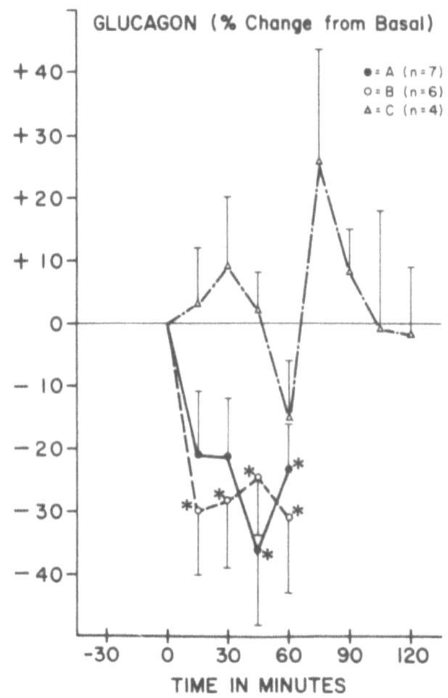

Figure 5. The effect of insulin therapy on the ability of glucose to suppress plasma glucagon concentrations in diabetic children. Group A are normal children infused with glucose. Group B are diabetic children pretreated with insulin prior to glucose infusion. Plasma glucagon falls significantly and, to a similar extent, in Group A and Group B. In contrast, diabetic children not treated with insulin (Group C) have no significant fall in glucagon during glucose infusion. [Data from Sperling et al. (1977b) by permission from the publishers].

the availability of insulin and supressibility of glucagon by glucose has been demonstrated (Buchanan and Mawhinney, 1973; Josefsberg, Laron, Doron, Keret, Belinski, and Weismann, 1975).

Amino acids stimulate glucagon secretion and, at the same time, stimulate insulin release (Blackard, Nelson, and Andrews, 1974; Muller *et al.*, 1974b; Pagliara, Stillings, Hover, Martin, and Matchinsky, 1974; Rocha, Faloona, and Unger, 1972; Wise, Hendler, and Felig, 1972). Despite the rise in insulin during amino acid ingestion or infusion, blood glucose rises. This rise in glucose, despite the rise in insulin and in the absence of ingested glucose, attests to the importance of glucagon in maintaining glucose homeostasis; in the absence of glucagon, a fall in glucose would be expected. While a number of amino acids stimulate glucagon (Rocha *et al.*, 1972), arginine (Blackard *et al.*, 1974) or alanine (Wise *et al.*, 1973a) are potent stimuli, and the latter is an important gluconeogenic precursor (Wise *et al.*, 1973a). The response to alanine in an isolated pancreas is depicted in Figure 6. A rapid spike of secretion is followed by a sustained plateau, the typical biphasic response. The magnitude of the response can be modulated by glucose. Thus, hyperglycemia blunts the glucagon response to amino acids, while hypoglycemia exaggerates this glucagon response (Blackard *et al.*, 1974; Pagliara *et al.*, 1974). Again, the hyperresponsiveness of glucagon secretion induced by amino acids in diabetics is attributable to insulin deficiency. Normal responsiveness can be restored with the provision of insulin through ongoing infusion designed to achieve euglycemia (Aronoff, Bennett, Rushforth, Miller, and Unger, 1976a, 1976b; Aronoff, Bennett, and Unger, 1977; Gerich, Lorenzi, Tsalikian, Bohannon, Schneider, Karam, and Forsham, 1976a; Gerich *et al.*, 1975a; Ohneda, Shoji, Horigome, and Yamagata, 1975).

Free fatty acids (FFA) also exert an influence on glucagon secretion in a manner analogous to glucose (Gerich, Langlois, Schneider, Karam, and Noacco, 1974; Quabbe, Ramek, and Luyckx, 1977). Thus, elevation of FFA lowers plasma glucagon values, whereas a fall in plasma FFA is associated with a rise in glucagon. The effects of glucose predominate over those of FFA, so that glucagon levels remain suppressed during hyperglycemia despite the presence of low FFA levels. High FFA levels also blunt the glucagon rise in response to arginine, but low FFA levels do not augment this glucagon response. It should be noted that the combination of hyperglycemia and high FFA augment insulin secretion while suppressing glucagon levels.

During triglyceride absorption following a fat meal glucagon also rises; this rise is more impressive in dog than in man (Bottger, Dobbs, Faloona, and Unger, 1973; Dobbs, Faloona, and Unger, 1975). Moreover, the signal for glucagon secretion appears to be an enteric hormone rather than the chylomicronemia, since direct

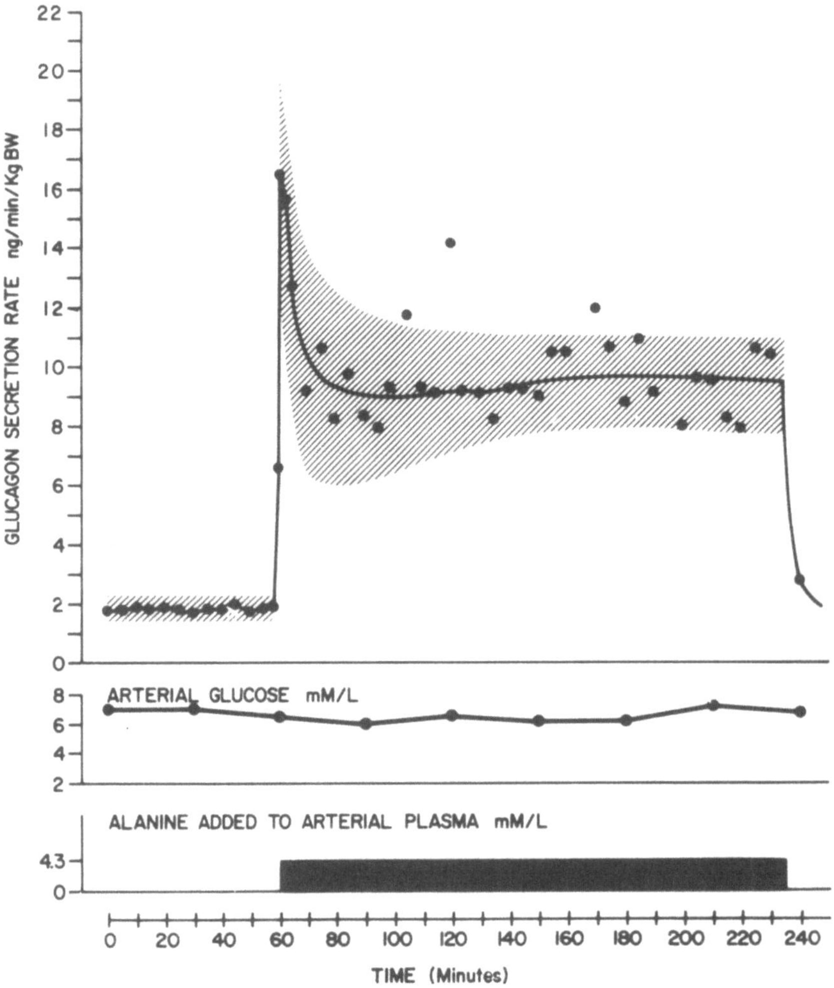

Figure 6. The effect of the amino acid alanine on glucagon secretion rate (GSR) in the isolated blood-perfused canine pancreas. There is a sharp spike followed by a sustained plateau of GSR during the alanine infusion. The shaded area represents the SEM around the mean depicted by the solid line of three studies.

intravenous infusion of chyle has no effect on glucagon levels (Bottger *et al.*, 1973). Although resistance to endogenous hyperglucagonemia has been invoked as one mechanism contributing to hypertriglyceridemia in certain experimental animals (Eaton and Schade, 1973; Tiengo, Muggeo, Assan, Fedele, and Crepaldi, 1975), the evidence in man does not appear to support this contention (Elkeles and Hambley, 1976).

Autonomic Influences on Glucagon Secretion

It has now been firmly established that epinephrine can stimulate glucagon secretion and that, like their neighbors the insulin secreting β-cells, the pancreatic α-cells are richly innervated with autonomic nerve endings that can modulate α-cell secretion (Woods and Porte, 1974). Direct electrical stimulation of the mixed autonomic nerves (Kaneto, Kajinuma, and Kosaka, 1975; Marliss, Girardier, Seydoux, Wollheim, Kanazawa, Orci, Renold, and Porte, 1973), direct infusion of epinephrine (Atkinson, Dahms, Sperling, and Bray, 1976; Gerich, Karam, and Forsham, 1973; Gerich, Langlois, Noacco, Schneider, and Forsham, 1974; Gerich, Lorenzi, Tsalikian, and Karam, 1976), exercise (Harvey, Faloona, and Unger, 1974; Luyckx and Lefebvre, 1974), trauma (Lindsey, Santeusanio, Braaten, Faloona, and Unger, 1974), and anxiety and stress (Bloom, Daniel, Johnston, Ogawa, and Pratt, 1972) stimulate glucagon secretion while simultaneously lowering insulin secretion. Similarly, the infusion or ingestion of L-dopa, a precursor of catecholamine biosynthesis stimulates glucagon secretion (Leblanc, Lachelin, Abu-Fadil, and Yey, 1977; Rayfield, George, Eichner, and Hsu, 1975). L-dopa and dopamine-stimulated glucagon secretion may not, however, be dependent on conversion to catecholamines, but may reflect the presence of dopaminergic nerve endings in the pancreas, particularly since L-dopa also stimulates insulin secretion rather than suppressing it. An unequivocal consensus as to whether α- or β-adrenergic receptors predominate in epinephrine-induced glucagon secretion has not been reached (Sperling and Voina, 1975). There is evidence that β-adrenergic agonists stimulate while α-adrenergic agonists suppress glucagon secretion. This view is not universally accepted and conflicting results have been reported using similar experimental protocols. Our own investigations suggest that both α- and β-adrenergic receptors are involved in glucagon secretion, as illustrated in Figure 7 (Atkinson *et al.*, 1976). This controversy should not obscure the importance of the fact that glucagon secretion is elevated in a number of stress states associated with high levels of catecholamines. Indeed, it has been demonstrated that the hyperglycemic effect of epinephrine is mediated, at least in part, through the stimulation of glucagon secretion (Gerich *et al.*, 1976). Other neurotransmitters may also be involved in modulating glucagon secretion; for example, serotonin appears to inhibit glucagon secretion (Marco, Hedo, Martinell, Calle, and Villanueva, 1976).

Parasympathetic

The parasympathetic nervous system, via stimulation of the vagus nerve and acetylcholine, also stimulates glucagon secretion whereas atropine or total vagotomy inhibit glucagon release (Bloom, Edwards, and Vaughan, 1974; Bloom and Vaughan, 1974; Iversen, 1973). Such diminished release of glucagon in totally vagotomized patients

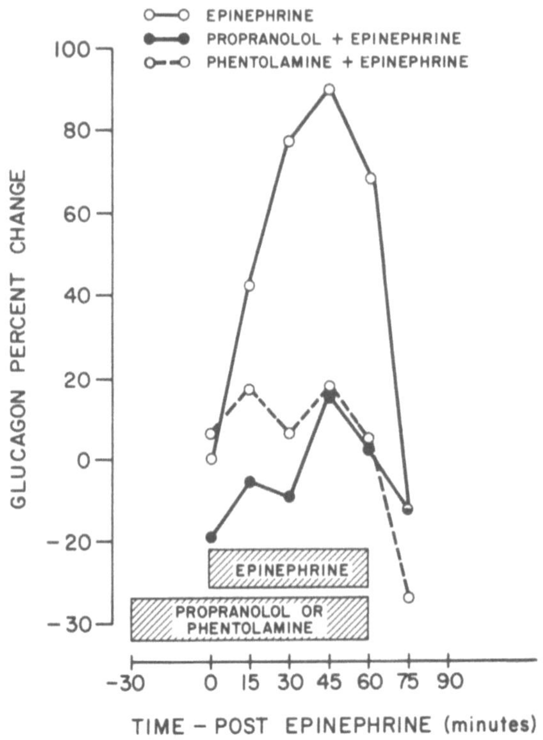

Figure 7. The effect of epinephrine with and without α-(phentolamine) of β-(propranolol) adrenergic blockade or plasma glucagon concentrations in man. The stimulation by epinephrine is prevented by both adrenergic blockers. [Adapted from Atkinson et al. (1976).]

may contribute to the observed reactive hypoglycemia following gastric surgery (Bloom and Vaughan, 1974). It has also been suggested that vagal activation during a fall in blood glucose would stimulate glucagon release and, hence, restore blood glucose levels to normal. Thus, the dual autonomic control of glucagon secretion is physiologically important; it would provide the means to restore glucose with impending hypoglycemia (parasympathetic) or elevate blood glucose during a variety of stress situations (sympathetic).

Miscellaneous Factors Affecting Glucagon Secretion

The factors affecting glucagon secretion are summarized in Table 1. In addition, there are a number of clinical conditions in which excessive glucagon secretion has been described (Table 2). These can be conveniently classified into endocrine disorders that include hyperparathyroidism, growth hormone excess, glucocorticoid excess, and pheochromocytoma, and miscellaneous conditions such as hepatic

Table 1. FACTORS AFFECTING GLUCAGON SECRETION

Nutrients	Ions	Hormones	Neurotransmitters
Glucose ↓	Calcium ↑	Insulin (hypoglycemia) ↑	Sympathetic ↑ Epinephrine Norepinephrine
Amino acids ↑	Potassium ↑	Growth hormone ↑	Parasympathetic ↑ Acetylcholine
Fatty acids ↓		Cortisol ↑	
		G.I. Hormones ↑ Secretin Gastrin Pancreozymin G.I.P.	Dopamine ↑ Serotonin ↓
		Local Somatostatin ↓ Prostaglandin ↑	

↑ *indicates that a rise in the factor stimulates glucagon release*

↓ *indicates that a rise in the factor inhibits glucagon release*

Table 2. MISCELLANEOUS CONDITIONS IN WHICH GLUCAGON IS ELEVATED

Acute pancreatitis
Hyperparathyroidism
Acromegaly
Cirrhosis
Pheochromocytoma
Glucocorticoid excess
Hyperlipoproteinemia

cirrhosis, renal failure, and pancreatitis. Neurotensin and prostaglandins also are capable of stimulating glucagon secretion. Calcium appears to be important in glucagon release, as it is for insulin release. Detailed discussion of each of these factors is beyond the scope of this review, the interested reader is referred to the cited references (Bhathena, Perrino, Voyles, Smith, Wilkins, Coy, Schally, and Recant, 1976; Bilbrey, Faloona, White, and Knochel, 1974; Curry and Bennett, 1974; Leclercq-Meyer, Marchand,

and Malaisse, 1973; Kuzuya, Kajinuma, and Ide, 1974; Ukai, Inoue, and Itatsu, 1977; Wise *et al.*, 1973b).

Glucagon Action

The primary effect of glucagon is to stimulate glycogenolysis via activation of adenyl cyclase, the formation of cAMP and the cascade that results in active liver phosphorylase breaking down glycogen (Sutherland and Robison, 1966). A second effect of glucagon is the stimulation of gluconeogenesis from amino acids; this effect takes longer to initiate but is of longer duration (Sokal, 1966). Thus, these two major effects of glucagon are to raise blood glucose concentration. As with other polypeptide hormones, glucagon action appears to be initiated by the binding to specific receptors on plasma membranes (Freychet, 1976; Phol, 1977). Unlike insulin, however, the data do not show a negative correlation between the circulating plasma concentration and the membrane binding of the hormone.

McGarry and Foster (1977) have recently suggested that glucagon is a key signal for hepatic ketogenesis. Using the rat as a model, they demonstrated that ketogenesis could be induced by anti-insulin antiserum, or by exposure of rats *in vivo* to glucagon concentrations within the high physiological range. Even in the presence of normal insulin levels, and with little change in peripheral glucose, FFA or ketone levels, the livers of glucagon-treated animals were capable of marked ketogenesis *in vitro*.

Glucagon's actions, therefore, are opposite to those of insulin and, with a few exceptions, glucagon secretion is stimulated at times when insulin secretion is inhibited and *vice versa*. Since both insulin and glucagon are secreted into the portal circulation and primarily act on the liver, it was suggested that the hepatic response in terms of anabolic effects mediated by insulin or catabolic effects mediated by glucagon was determined by the molar ratio of the two hormones rather than by the absolute concentration of each (Unger, 1971). Support for this hypothesis was strengthened by showing that hepatic glucose output remained constant over a 100-fold range in the concentration of glucagon and insulin provided that the ratio of the two hormones remained constant (Parrilla, Goodman, and Toews, 1974). Thus, the two islet hormones, insulin and glucagon, appeared to act as a push-pull system to finely regulate hepatic glucose output or uptake and, thereby, control the disposition of exogenous or endogenous nutrient according to the "need" for glucose, or other energy sources.

Glucagon in the Newborn Period

One time of nutrient need is the immediate newborn period when the nutrient supply to the fetus is dramatically curtailed with separation of the placenta. Studies from our laboratory, as well as others, have demonstrated that in human newborns or the newborns of sheep, rat, and rabbit, there is a dramatic surge in glucagon within hours of birth while insulin remains low (Grajwer, Sperling, Sack, and Fisher, 1977; Sperling, DeLamater, Phelps, Fisher, Oh, and Fisher, 1972). Such a hormonal profile would tend to initiate glycogenolysis as well as ketogenesis and, possibly, gluconeogenesis, arrest the fall in glucose, and provide glucose for brain metabolism and ketones as alternate fuel for muscle metabolism. Interestingly, this glucagon surge is deficient in infants born to diabetic mothers and these infants are prone to the development of hypoglycemia (Williams, Sperling, and Racasa, 1975). The importance of glucagon in the neonatal period is further supported through studies with somatostatin (SRIF). When SRIF is infused to newborn lambs, aged one to three days, there is a fall in both glucagon and insulin and a significant fall in glucose. With ongoing SRIF infusion of glucagon at physiological concentrations resotres glucose toward normal, whereas infusion of insulin while glucagon is low results in profound hypoglycemia (Sperling, Grajwar, Leake, and Fisher, 1977c).

Significance of Glucagon Secretion and Action

In normal fasting man, acute infusion of SRIF results in a fall in glucose when both insulin and glucagon are suppressed. Reinfusion of glucagon, while insulin remains suppressed, results in hyperglycemia (Gerich, Lorenzi, Hane, Gustafson, Guillemin, and Forsham, 1975c). It should be noted that in all forms of experimentally induced or spontaneous diabetes in animals or man where insulin is deficient, there is relative glucagon excess, *i.e.*, glucagon is inappropriately high for the prevaling blood glucose level, cannot be suppressed by additional glucose in the absence of insulin, and usually there is hypersecretion of glucagon in response to stimuli such as amino acids (Dobbs, Sakurai, Sasaki, Faloona, Valverde, Baetens, Orci, and Unger, 1975b; Sakurai, Dobbs, and Unger, 1976). Thus, the proposition of Unger *et al.* that glucagon was essential for the hyperglycemia of diabetes had considerable appeal based on documented observations (Unger and Orci, 1975).

If the hypothesis concerning the importance of glucagon as a key factor in the genesis of hyperglycemia and ketonemia in diabetes were correct, then suppression of glucagon secretion should result in amelioration of these findings or in delayed development of hyperglycemia and ketonemia when insulin was withheld. The results of initial investigations strongly supported this hypothesis. Thus, the infusion of SRIF in insulin-dependent diabetics markedly blunted a meal-induced rise in glucagon and in glucose (Gerich, Lorenzi, Schneider, Karam, Rivier, Guillemin, and Forsham, 1974d). The combination of SRIF, together with insulin, actually caused a fall in blood glucose despite the ingested meal. Moreover, a prolonged (18 hour) infusion of SRIF in diabetic patients deprived of insulin markedly delayed the appearance and severity of hyperglycemia and of hyperglucagonemia, as well as that of ketosis, when compared to the same subjects infused with saline only (Gerich, Lorenzi, Bier, Schneider, Tsalikian, Karam, and Forsham, 1975b). Also, the insulin requirement in insulin-dependent diabetics treated by a computerized insulin delivery system, the so-called artificial pancreas, was reduced by as much as 60% when SRIF was simultaneously infused (Meissner, Thum, Beischer, Winkler, Schroder, and Pfeiffer, 1975). Even in the absence of SRIF infusion, when insulin was withheld from diabetics, the rise in glucagon and the rises in FFA and ketone bodies were significantly correlated (Alberti, Christensen, Iversen, and Orskov, 1975). It should be noted, however, that once well established, diabetic ketoacidosis can not be reversed by infusion of SRIF alone, although glucose concentrations do fall (Lundbaek, Christensen, Hansen, Iversen, Orskow, and Seyer-Hansen, 1976).

More recently this hypothesis has been challenged by the following observations. Firstly, diabetic ketoacidosis will develop in insulin-deprived pancreatectomized subjects in whom glucagon levels are extremely low and in whom no further increment in glucagon occurs following stimulation with arginine (Barnes and Bloom, 1976; Barnes *et al.*, 1977). It must be emphasized that the rate of development of diabetic ketoacidosis is markedly delayed, that the plasma levels of glucose and ketones are significantly lower, and that the dose of insulin required to maintain glucose homeostasis is significantly less than in the usual insulin-dependent diabetic. What is challenged, therefore, is the concept of the essentiality of glucagon for the development of the metabolic abnormalities; glucagon clearly contributes to the rate, accelerating the development of diabetic ketoacidosis.

Second is the issue whether the abnormalities in glucagon secretion are a primary disturbance, or secondary to insulin deficiency. Restoration of normal glucagon responsiveness to stimulation or glucose suppression by the appropriate use of insulin has now been demonstrated by a number of investigators, including early proponents of the concept that disturbance in glucagon secretion in diabetes was primary. And no abnormality in glucagon secretion has been observed in prediabetes as long as insulin secretion is normal. Thus, the hyperglucagonemia of diabetes appears to be secondary to insulin deficiency, as would appear to be the case for growth hormone (Sperling, 1977a).

Thirdly, the infusion of glucagon at doses which achieve plasma concentrations of 300 to 700 *pg/mℓ*, *i.e.*, concentrations found in the portal vein or in peripheral plasma during diabetic ketoacidosis, does not alter glucose levels during an oral glucose tolerance test. It also does not alter the daily profiles of glucose in maturity onset diabetes, nor in juvenile diabetes providing that insulin is given. In the absence of given insulin, the hyperglycemic effect of glucagon is quite pronounced. Thus, as long as insulin is available the effect of glucagon appears to be minor (Sherwin, Fisher, Hendler, and Felig, 1976). Furthermore, patients who harbor a glucagonoma, usually have mild, noninsulin-dependent diabetes (Mallison, Bloom, Warin, Salmon, and Cox, 1974).

Fourthly, it was demonstrated that SRIF reduces splanchnic blood flow and delays the absorption of carbohydrate, including xylose. These effects cannot be reversed by the infusion of glucagon. Thus, the postprandial glucose-lowering effect of SRIF appears to be due to delayed absorption rather than to suppression of glucagon. Conversely, the postprandial hyperglycemia of diabetes appears to be primarily the result of insulin deficiency rather than glucagon excess (Wahren and Felig, 1976).

Fifthly, during prolonged SRIF infusion, glucagon and insulin remain suppressed throughout. Glucose, on the other hand, initially falls, but, after two to three hours of SRIF infusion, rises steadily despite low glucagon levels, suggesting that the effects of insulin deficiency are becoming manifest. Furthermore, when SRIF infusion is discontinued, there is a rebound rise in glucagon and insulin; despite the rise in glucagon, glucose falls, reflecting the effects of the rising insulin. Thus, it could be anticipated that in normal subjects, or in patients with maturity onset diabetes and residual insulin-secreting capacity, prolonged infusion of SRIF would result in an initial fall of glucose followed by the development or exacerbation of diabetes. This is, indeed, the case, as recently demonstrated in independent studies from two different groups (Tamborlane, Sherwin, Hendler, and Felig, 1977; Waldhausl, Bratusch-Marrain, Dudczak, and Deutsch, 1977). The use of SRIF alone, in the absence of the provision of some insulin, is therefore strongly contraindicated.

How can one reconcile these powerful arguments against the importance of glucagon (Barnes, Bloom, Crowley, Tuttlebee, Bloom, Alberti, Smythe, and Turnell, 1975) with equally convincing early data? In the course of studies wherein glucagon was constantly infused at physiological concentrations, it was noted that, in normal subjects, the rise in peripheral blood glucose was transient, returning to baseline values within one hour despite ongoing glucagon infusion. A transient rise in insulin levels was also observed (Sherwin *et al.*, 1976). Further studies established that the brief change in peripheral blood glucose was due to an equally brief rise in hepatic glucose output (Bomboy *et al.*, 1977; Bomboy, Jr. *et al.*, 1977; Cherrington *et al.*, 1976; Felig *et al.*, 1976; Felig *et al.*,

1975). This brief rise in hepatic glucose output was not dependent on insulin as it was also observed in insulin-deprived diabetic subjects or animals (Bomboy *et al.*, 1977; Bomboy, Jr. *et al.*, 1977; Cherrington *et al.*, 1976; Felig *et al.*, 1976; Felig *et al.*, 1975). In the absence of insulin, however, the brief rise in hepatic glucose output resulted in a pronounced rise in peripheral blood glucose, reflecting the importance of insulin for peripheral metabolism of glucose (Sherwin *et al.*, 1976). The mechanism responsible for the diminished hepatic glucose output in the face of ongoing glucagon infusion remains unknown.

The techniques of measuring hepatic glucose output, coupled with the ability to produce selective deficiency of insulin or glucagon via infusion of SRIF, have enabled the documentation of the real contribution of glucagon to glucose homeostasis (Cherrington *et al.*, 1976). In the absence of glucagon, glucose production declines about one-third from basal; glucagon reinfusion restores basal glucose production. In the absence of insulin, basal glucagon concentrations augment glucose production by some 50% above basal. Thus, each of these pancreatic hormones has an important role in regulating hepatic glucose output, and the absence of either glucagon or insulin results, respectively, in under- or overproduction (Cherrington *et al.*, 1976). Although the liver becomes refractory to a constant infusion of glucagon so that hepatic glucose output returns to the basal level, this basal rate of glucose production is now dependent on this new high concentration of glucagon. A sudden interruption in the rate of glucagon infusion results in a dramatic fall in glucose production and in peripheral hypoglycemia (Shulman, Williams, Lacy, and Cherrington, 1977). As long as glucagon infusion is ongoing, the rate of gluconeogenesis continues to increase so that, although total hepatic glucose output returns to basal levels, the proportion emanating from gluconeogenesis increases (Schulman *et al.*, 1977).

These recent observations again suggest that both glucagon and insulin are key hormones in regulating hepatic glucose output (Bomboy *et al.*, 1977; Bomboy Jr. *et al.* 1977; Cherrington *et al.*, 1976; Felig *et al.*, 1976; Felig *et al.*, 1975; Schulman *et al.*, 1977), and that, in normal man, the acute changes in either hormone act as an efficient control system to prevent wide fluctuations in glucose levels thereby maintaining an exquisite control of glucose homeostasis. In insulin-dependent diabetes, the primary abnormality is insulin deficiency resulting in secondary elevations in glucagon. Hyperglucagonemia accelerates the metabolic abnormalities of diabetes that are due to insulin deficiency, and that consequently cannot be prevented by suppression of glucagon alone. Therefore, therapy for diabetes must focus primarily on means to provide insulin in a manner which will simulate as closely as possible normal events and, secondarily, maintain normal or low glucagon concentrations. At the same time, in resolving some of the controversies regarding glucagon, ongoing research is uncovering newer aspects which increase our understanding of normal and abnormal physiology. One newer aspect will be the elucidation of the mechanism responsible for the transient effect of glucagon on hepatic glucose output.

ACKNOWLEDGEMENTS

I gratefully acknowledge the skilled secretarial assistance of Ms. Joy Reynolds and the stimulating advice of colleagues and fellows, without whom this paper and our own results reported herein would not be possible.

REFERENCES

Aguilar-Parada, E., Eisentraut, A., and Unger, R.H. 1969. Effects of starvation on plasma pancreatic glucagon in normal man. *Diabetes* **18**:717-723.

Alberti, K.G.M.M., Christensen, N.J., Iversen, J., and Orskov, H. 1975. Role of glucagon and other hormones in development of diabetic ketoacidosis. *Lancet* I:1307-1311.

Alford, F.P., Bloom, S.R., and Nabarro, J.D.M. 1977. Glucagon levels in normal and diabetic subjects: Use of a specific immunoabsorbent for glucagon radioimmunoassay. *Diabetologia* **13**:1-6.

Aronoff, S.L., Bennett, P.H., Rushforth, N.B., Miller, M., and Unger, R. 1976a. Arginine-stimulated hyperglucagonemia in diabetic Pima Indians. *Diabetes* **25**:404-407.

Aronoff, S.L., Bennett, P.H., Rushforth, N.B., Miller, M., and Unger, R.H. 1976b. Normal glucagon response to arginine infusion in "prediabetic" Pima Indians. *J. Clin. Endocrinol. Metab.* **43**:279-286.

Aronoff, S.L., Bennett, P.H., and Unger R.H. 1977. Immunoreactive glucagon (IRG) responses to intravenous glucose in prediabetes and diabetes among Pima Indians and normal Caucasians. *J. Clin, Endocrinol. Metab.* **44**:968-972.

Atkinson, R.L., Dahms, W.T., Sperling, M.A., and Bray, G.A. 1976. Adrenergic modulation of glucagon secretion in obese humans. *Endocrine Society Program of 58th Annual Meeting*, p. 303. (Abstr.)

Barnes, A.H. and Bloom, S.R. 1976. Pancreatectomized man: A model for diabetes without glucagon. *Lancet* I:219-221.

Barnes, A.J., Bloom, S.T., Alberti, K.G.M.M., Smythe, P., Alford, F.P., and Chishold, D.J. 1977. Ketoacodosis in pancreatectomized man. *New Eng. J. Med.* **296**:1250-1253.

Barnes, A.J., Bloom, A., Crowley, M.F., and Tuttlebee, J.W. 1975. Is glucagon important in stable insulin-dependent diabetics? *Lancet* II:734-737.

Bhathena, S.J., Perrino, P.V., Voyles, N.R., Smith, S.S., Wilkins, S.D., Coy, D.H., Schally, A.V., and Recant, L. 1976. Reversal of somatostatin inhibition of insulin and glucagon secretion. *Diabetes* **25**:1031-1040.

Bilbrey, G.L., Faloona, G.R., White, M.G., and Knochel, J.P. 1974. Hyperglucagonemia of renal failure. *J. Clin. Invest.* **53**:841-847.

Blackard, W.G., Nelson, N.C., and Andrews, S.S. 1974. Portal and peripheral vein immunoreactive glucagon concentrations after arginine or glucose infusions. *Diabetes* **23**:199-202.

Bloom, S.R., Daniel, P.M., Johnston, D.I., Ogawa, O., and Pratt, O.E. 1972. Changes in glucagon level associated with anxiety or stress. *Psychol. Med.* **2**:426-427.

Bloom, S.R., Edwards, A.V., and Vaughan, N.J.A. 1974a. The role of the autonomic innervation in the control of glucagon release during hypoglycemia in the calf. *J. Physiol.* **236**:611-623.

Bloom, S.R., Vaughan, N.J.A., and Russel, R.C.G. 1974b. Vagal control of glucagon release in man. *Lancet* **II**:546-549.

Boden, G. and Owen, O.E. 1977. Familial hyperglucagonemia--an autosomal dominant disorder. *New Eng. J. Med.* **296**:534-538.

Bomboy, J.E., Lewis, S.B., Lacy, W.W., Sinclair-Smith, B.C., and Liljenquist, J.E. 1977b. Transient stimulatory effect of sustained hyperglucagonemia on splanchnic glucose production in normal and diabetic man. *Diabetes* **26**:177-184.

Bomboy, J.E., Jr., Lewis, S.B., Sinclair-Smith, B.C., Lacy, W.W., and Liljenquist, J.E. 1977a. Insulin-glucagon interaction in controlling splanchnic glucose production in normal man. *J. Clin. Endocrinol. Metab.* **44**:474-480.

Bottger, I., Dobbs, R., Faloona, G.R., and Unger, R.H. 1973. The effects of triglyceride absorption upon glucagon, insulin, and gut glucagon-like immunoreactivity. *J. Clin. Invest.* **52**:2532-2541.

Bratten, J.T., Faloona, G.R., and Unger, R.H. 1974. The effect of insulin on the *alpha*-cell response to hyperglycemia in long-standing alloxan diabetes. *J. Clin. Invest.* **53**:1017-1021.

Buchanan, K.D. and Mawhinney, A.A. 1973. Insulin control of glucagon release from insulin-deficient rat islets. *Diabetes* **22**:801-803.

Cherrington, S.A., Chiasson, J.L., Liljenquist, J.E., Jennings, A.S., Keller, U., and Lacy, W.W. 1976. The role of insulin and glucagon in the regulation of basal glucose production in the postabsorptive dog. *J. Clin, Invest.* **58**:1407-1418.

Curry, D.L. and Bennett, L.L. 1974. Reversal of somatostatin inhibition of insulin secretion by calcium. *Biochem. Biophys. Res. Commun.* **60**:1015-1019.

Dobbs, R., Faloona, G.R., and Unger, R.H. 1975a. Effect of intravenously administered glucose on glucagon and insulin secretion during fat absorption. *Metabolism* **24**:69-75.

Dobbs, R., Sakurai, H., Sasaki, H., Faloona, G., Valverde, I., Baetens, D., Orci, L., and Unger, R. 1975b. Glucagon: Role in the hyperglycemia of diabetes mellitus. *Science* **187**:544-547.

Eaton, R.P. and Schade, D.S. 1973. Glucagon resistance as a hormonal basis for endogenous hyperlipaemia. *Lancet* I:973-974.

Elkeles, R.S. and Hambley, J. 1976. Glucagon resistance as a cause of hypertriglyceridemia. *Lancet* II:18-19.

Felig, P., Wahren, J., and Hendler, R. 1976a. Influence of physiologic hyperglucagonemia on basal and insulin-inhibited splanchnic glucose output in normal man. *J. Clin. Invest.* 58:761-765.

Felig, P., Wahren, J., Sherwin, R., and Hendler, R. 1975b. Insulin, glucagon, and somatostatin in normal physiology and diabetes mellitus. *Diabetes* 25:1091-1099.

Freychet, P. 1976. Interactions of polypeptide hormones with cell membrane specific receptors: Studies with insulin and glucagon. *Diabetologia* 12:83-100.

Gabbay, K.H., DeLuca, K., Fisher, J.N., Mako, M.E., and Rubenstein, A.H. 1976. Familial hyperproinsulinemia: An autosomal dominant defect. *New Eng. J. Med.* 294:911-915.

Gerich, J.E., Karam, J.H., and Forsham, P.H. 1973. Stimulation of glucagon secretion by epinephrine in man. *J. Clin. Endocrinol. Metab.* 37:479-481.

Gerich, J.E., Langlois, M., Noacco, C., Schneider, F., and Forsham, P.H. 1974c. Adrenergic modulation of pancreatic glucagon secretion in man. *J. Clin. Invest.* 53:1441-1446.

Gerich, J.E., Langlois, M., Schneider, F., Karam, J.H., and Noacco, C. 1974b. Effects of alterations of plasma free fatty acid levels on pancreatic glucagon secretion in man. *J. Clin. Invest.* 53:1284-1289.

Gerich, J.E., Lorenzi, M., Bier, D.M., Schneider, V., Tsalikian, E., Karam, J.H., and Forsham, P.H. 1975b. Prevention of human diabetic ketoacidosis by somatostatin: Evidence for an essential role of glucagon. *New Eng. J. Med.* 292:985-989.

Gerich, J.E., Lorenzi, M., Hane, S., Gustafson, G., Guillemin, R., and Forsham, P.H. 1975c. Evidence for a physiologic role of pancreatic glucagon in human glucose homeostasis: Studies with somatostatin. *Metabolism* 24:175-182.

Gerich, J.E., Lorenzi, M., Schneider, V., Karam, J.H., Rivier, J., Guillemin, R., and Forsham, P.H. 1974d. Effects of somatostatin on plasma glucose and glucagon levels in human diabetes mellitus: Pathophysiologic and therapeutic implications. *New Eng. J. Med.* 291:544-547.

Gerich, J.E., Lorenzi, M., Tsalikian, E., Bohannon, N.V., Schneider, V., Karam, J.H., and Forsham, P.H. 1976a. Effects of acute insulin withdrawal and administration on plasma glucagon responses to intravenous arginine in insulin-dependent diabetic subjects. *Diabetes* 25:955-960.

Gerich, J.E., Lorenzi, M., Tsalikian, E., and Karam, J.H. 1976b. Studies on the mechanism of epinephrine-induced hyperglycemia in man: Evidence for participation of pancreatic glucagon secretion. *Diabetes* 25:65-71.

Gerich, J.E., Schneider, V., Dippe, S.E., Langlois, M., Noacco, C., Karam, J.H., and Forsham, P.H. 1974a. Characterization of the glucagon response to hypoglycemia in man. *J. Clin. Endocrinol. Metab.* **38**:77-82.

Gerich, J.E., Tsalikian, E., Lorenzi, M., Schneider, V., Bohannon, N.V., Gustafson, G., and Karam, J.H. 1975a. Normalization of fasting hyperglucagonemia and excessive glucagon responses to intravenous arginine in human diabetes mellitus by prolonged infusion of insulin. *J. Clin. Endocrinol. Metab.* 41:1178-1180.

Grajwer, L.A., Sperling, M.A., Sack, J., and Fisher, D.A. 1977. Possible mechanisms and significance of the neonatal surge in glucagon secretion: Studies in newborn lambs. *Pediat. Res.* 11:833-836.

Harvey, W.D., Faloona, C.R., and Unger, R.H. 1974. The effect of adrenergic blockade on exercise-induced hyperglucagonemia. *Endocrinology* **94**:1254-1258.

Iversen, J. 1973. Effect of acetylcholine on the secretion of glucagon and insulin from the isolated, perfused canine pancreas. *Diabetes* 22:381-387.

Josefsberg, Z., Laron, Z., Doron, M., Keret, R., Belinski, Y., and Weisman, I. 1975. Plasma glucagon response to arginine infusion in children and adolescents with diabetes mellitus. *Clin. Endocrinol.* **4**:487-492.

Kaneto, A., Kajinuma, H., and Kosaka, K. 1975. Effect of splanchnic nerve stimulation on glucagon and insulin output in the dog. *Endocrinology* **96**:143-150.

Kuku, S.F., Zeidler, A., Emmanouel, D.S., Katz, A.I., and Rubenstein, A.H. 1976. Heterogeneity of plasma glucagon: Patterns in patients with chronic renal failure and diabetes. *J. Clin. Endocrinol. Metab.* 42:173-176.

Kuzuya, T., Kajinuma, H., and Ide, T. 1974. Effect of intrapancreatic injection of potassium and calcium on insulin and glucagon secretion in dogs. *Diabetes* **23**:55-60.

Lawrence, A.M., Tan, S., Hojvat, S., and Kirsteins, L. 1977. Salivary gland hyperglycemic factor: An extrapancreatic source of glucagon-like material. *Science* 195:70-72.

Leblanc, H., Lachelin, G.C.L., Abu-Fadil, S. and Yen, S.C. 1977. The effect of dopamine infusion on insulin and glucagon secretion in man. *J. Clin. Endocrinol. Metab.* **44**:196-198.

Leclercq-Meyer, V., Marchand, J., and Malaisse, W.J. 1973. The effect of calcium and magnesium on glucagon secretion. *Endocrinology* **93**:1360-1370.

Lindsey, A., Santeusanio, F., Braaten, J., Faloona, G.R., and Unger, R.H. 1974. Pancreatic *alpha*-cell function in trauma. *J. Am. Med. Assoc.* **227**:757-761.

Lundbaek, K., Christensen, S.E., Hansen, A.P., Iversen, J., Orskov, H., and Seyer-Hansen, K. 1976. Failure of somatostatin to correct manifest diabetic ketoacidosis. *Lancet* I:215-218.

Luyckx, A. and Lefebvre, P.J. 1974. Mechanisms involved in the exercise-induced increase in glucagon secretion in rats. *Diabetes* 23:81-93.

McGarry, J.D. and Foster, D.W. 1977. Hormonal control of ketogenesis. *Arch. Intern. Med.* 137:495-501.

Mallison, C.N., Bloom, S.R., Warin, A.P., Salmon, P.R., and Cox, B. 1974. A glucagonoma syndrome. *Lancet* II:1-5.

Marco, J., Hedo, J.A., Martinell, J., Calle, C., and Villeanueva, M.L. 1976. Potentiation of glucagon secretion by serotonin antagonists in man. *J. Clin. Endocrinol. Metab.* 42:215-221.

Marliss, E.B., Girardier, L., Seydoux, J., Wollheim, C.B., Kanazawa, Y., Orci, L., Renold, A.E., and Porte, D., Jr. 1973. Glucagon release induced by pancreatic nerve stimulation in the dog. *J. Clin. Invest.* 52:1246-1259.

Matsuyama, T., Hoffman, W.H., Dunbar, J.C., Foa, N.L., and Foa, P.P. 1976. Glucose, insulin, pancreatic glucagon and glucagon-like immunoreactive materials in the plasma of normal and diabetic children. Effect of the initial insulin treatment. *Horm. Metab. Res.* 7:451-456.

Meissner, C., Thum, C.H., Beischer, W., Winkler, G., Schroder, K.E., and Pfeiffer, E.F. 1975. Antidiabetic action of somatostatin--Assessed by the artificial pancreas. *Diabetes* 24:988-996.

Muller, W.A., Faloona, G.R., and Unger, R.H. 1971a. The effect of experimental insulin deficiency on glucagon secretion. *J. Clin. Invest.* 50:1992-1999.

Muller, W.A., Faloona, G.R., and Unger, R.H. 1971b. The effect of alanine on glucagon secretion. *J. Clin. Invest.* 50:2215-2218.

Ohneda, A., Ishii, S., Horigome, K., and Yamagata, S. 1975. Glucagon response to arginine after treatment of diabetes mellitus. *Diabetes* 24:811-819.

Pagliara, A.S., Stillings, S.N., Hover, B., Martin, D.M., and Matschinsky, F.M. 1974. Glucose modulation of amino acid-induced glucagon and insulin release in the isolated perfused rat pancreas. *J. Clin. Invest.* 54:819-832.

Palmer, J.P. and Ensinck, J.W. 1974. Stimulation of glucagon secretion by ethanol-induced hypoglycemia in man. *Diabetes* 24:295-300.

Parrilla, R., Goodman, M.N., and Toews, C.J. 1974. Effect of glucagon:insulin ratios on hepatic metabolism. *Diabetes* 23:725-731.

Pohl, S.L. 1977. The glucagon receptor and its relationship to adenylate cyclase. *Fed. Proc.* 36:2115-2118.

Quabbe, H.G., Ramek, W., and Luyckx, A.S. 1977. Growth hormone, glucagon, and insulin response to depression of plasma free fatty acids and the effect of glucose infusion. *J. Clin.*

Endocrinol. Metab. 44:383.
Raskin, R., Fujita, Y., and Unger, R.H. 1975. Effect of insulin-glucose infusions on plasma glucagon levels in fasting diabetics and non-diabetics. *J. Clin. Invest.* **36**:1132-1138.
Rayfield, E.J., George, D.T., Eichner, H.L., and Hsu, T.H. 1975. L-dopa stimulation of glucagon secretion in man. *New Eng. J. Med.* **293**:589-591.
Rocha, D.M., Faloona, G.R., and Unger, R.H. 1972. Glucagon-stimulating activity of 20 amino acids in dogs. *J. Clin. Invest.* **51**:2346-2351.
Sakurai, H., Dobbs, R.E., and Unger, R.H. 1975. The role of glucagon in the pathogenesis of the endogenous hyperglycemia of diabetes mellitus. *Metabolism* **24**:1287-1297.
Sasaki, H., Rubalcave, B., Baetens, D., Blazquez, E., Srikant, C.B., Orci, L., and Unger, R.H. 1975. Identification of glucagon in the gastrointestinal tract. *J. Clin. Invest.* **56**:135-145.
Schulman, G.I., Williams, P.E., Lacy, W.W., and Cherrington, A.D. 1977. Adaptation of glucose production to a physiological increment in glucagon. *Diabetes* **26** (Suppl. 1):383. (Abstr.)
Sherwin, R.S., Fisher, M., Hendler, R., and Felig, P. 1976. Glucagon and glucose regulation in normal, obese and diabetic subjects. *New Eng. J. Med.* **294**:455-462.
Sokal, J.E. 1966. Effect of glucagon on gluconeogenesis by the isolated perfused rat liver. *Endocrinology* **78**:537-548.
Sperling, M.A. 1977. The contribution of hyperglycemic hormones to the pathogenesis of diabetes mellitus. *Am. J. Dis. Child.* **131**:1145-1149.
Sperling, M.A., Aleck, K., and Voina, S. 1977. Suppressibility of glucagon secretion by glucose in juvenile diabetes. *J. Pediatr.* **90**:543-547.
Sperling, M.A., DeLamater, P.V., Kazenelson, M., Fiser, R.H., and Fisher, D. 1974. Development and application of a radioimmunoassay for plasma glucagon. *Clin. Chem.* **20**:566-570.
Sperling, M.A., DeLamater, P.V., Phelps, D., Riser, R.H., Oh, K., and Fisher, D.A. 1974. Spontaneous and amino acid-stimulated glucagon secretion in the immediate postnatal period: Relation to glucose and insulin. *J. Clin. Invest.* **53**:1159-1166.
Sperling, M.A., Grajwer, L., Leake, R.D., and Fisher, D.A. 1977. Effects of somatostatin (SRIF) infusion on glucose homeostasis in newborn lambs. Evidence for a significant role of glucagon. *Pediatr. Res.* **11**:962-967.
Sperling, M.A. and Voina, S. 1975. Effect of adrenergic blockade on glucagon and growth hormone secretion in normal and diabetic children. *Pediatr. Res.* **9**:748-752.
Srikant, C.B., McCorkle, K., and Unger, R.H. 1977. Properties of immunoreactive glucagon fractions of canine stomach and pancreas. *J. Biol. Chem.* **252**:1846-1851.
Sundby, F., Jacobsen, H., and Moody, A.J. 1976. Purification and characterization of a protein from porcine gut with glucagon-like immunoreactivity. *Horm. Metab. Res.* **8**:366-371.

Sutherland, E.W. and Robison, G.A. 1966. The role of cyclic 3', 5'-AMP in responses to catecholamines and other hormones. *Pharmacol. Rev.* **18**:145-161.

Tamborlane, W.V., Sherwin, R.S., Hendler, R., and Felig, P. 1977. Metabolic effects of somatostatin in maturity-onset diabetes. *New Eng. J. Med.* **297**:181-183.

Tiengo, A., Muggeo, M., Assan, R., Fedele, D., and Crepaldi, G. 1975. Glucagon secretion in primary endogenous hypertriglyceridemia before and after clofibrate treatment. *Metabolism* 24:901-914.

Ukai, M., Inoue, I., and Tatsu, T. 1977. Effect of somatostatin on neurotensin-induced glucagon release and hyperglycemia. *Endocrinology* **100**:1284-1286.

Unger, R.H. 1971. Glucagon and the insulin:glucagon ratio in diabetes and other catabolic illnesses. *Diabetes* **20**:834-838.

Unger, R.H. 1974. *Alpha*- and *beta*-cell interrelationships in health and disease. *Metabolism* **23**:581-593.

Unger, R.H., Aguilar-Parada, E., Muller, W.A., and Eisentraut, A.M. 1970. Studies of pancreatic *alpha* cell function in normal and diabetic subjects. *J. Clin. Invest.* **49**:837-848.

Unger, R.H. and Orci, L. 1975. The essential role of glucagon in the pathogenesis of diabetes mellitus. *Lancet* **I**:14-16.

Vale, W., Brazeau, P., Rivier, C., Brown, M., Boss, B., Rivier, J., Burgus, R., Ling, N., and Guillemin, R. 1975. Somatostatin. *Recent Prog. Horm. Res.* 365-397.

Valverde, I., Dobbs, R., and Unger, R.H. 1975. Heterogeneity of plasma glucagon immunoreactivity in normal, depancreatized, and alloxan-diabetic dogs. *Metabolism* **24**:1021-1028.

Wahren, J. and Felig, P. 1976. Influence of somatostatin on carbohydrate disposal and absorption in diabetes mellitus. *Lancet* II:1213-1216.

Waldhausl, W., Bratusch-Marrain, P., Dudczak, R., and Deutsch, E. 1977. The diabetogenic action of somatostatin in healthy subjects and in maturity onset diabetics. *J. Clin. Endocrinol. Metab.* 44:876-883.

Williams, P,R., Sperling, M.A., and Racasa, Z. 1975. Blunting of spontaneous and amino acid stimulated glucagon secretion in infants of diabetic mothers. *Diabetes* **24** (Suppl. 2):411.

Wise, J.K., Hendler, R., and Felig, P. 1973a. Evaluation of *alpha*-cell function by infusion of alanine in normal, diabetic and obese subjects. *New Eng. J. Med.* **288**:484-487.

Wise, J.K., Hendler, R., and Felig, P. 1973b. Influence of glucocorticoids on glucagon secretion and plasma amino acid concentrations in man. *J. Clin. Invest.* **52**:2774-2782.

Woods, S.C. and Porte, D. 1974. Neural control of the endocrine pancreas. *Psychol. Rev.* **54**:596-619.

DISCUSSION FOLLOWING DR. SPERLING'S TALK

Dr. Burns

Thank you very much, Dr. Sperling, for a very lucid and comprehensive review of the glucagon story.

Dr. Ivey

I am interested in the gastric effects of glucagon. In view of the fact that glucagon inhibits gastric secretion in man and animals, can you postulate a physiological effect for glucagon in gastric physiology?

Dr. Sperling

Well, that degree of physiology is not known. I think, as Dr. Levine pointed out yesterday, the next major exciting step in the understanding of the metabolic effects of these hormones is going to be the unraveling of the interrelationships between glucagon, insulin, and somatostatin as an interrelating system, with glucagon being able to stimulate insulin, insulin being responsible for the normal suppression of glucagon, and somatostatin being responsible for the suppression of both insulin and glucagon. We also need to consider that glucagon appears to be a key stimulus to somatostatin secretion, and then the data that somatostatin seems to inhibit splanchnic blood flow and at the same time inhibit absorption--whether this process is because of the diminished splanchnic blood flow or a separate mechanism, I don't think has been totally defined yet. So the interrelationship of these hormones, these GI hormones if you will, produced by the pancreas which may be considered a vestigial organ from the embryological gut, is going to be important in terms of understanding normal physiology and normal digestion and absorption.

One could propose, for example, that under normal circumstances the ingestion of a meal results in the stimulation of somatostatin secretion; that somatostatin secretion, as a result of the rapid absorption of glucose, inhibits the rate of glucose entry; and that somatostatin, therefore, might be responsible in part for the normal pattern of blood glucose that one observes during the glucose tolerance test. The stimulation of somatostatin secretion may be responsible, in part, for the fall in insulin secretion that one observes, the initial rise and then the fall, as well as for the fall in glucagon secretion.

Dr. Ivey
What effect does gastrin have on glucagon?

Dr. Sperling
Gastrin stimulates glucagon secretion and, conversely, glucagon stimulates gastrin secretion.

Dr. Ivey
You said that somatostatin decreases xylose absorption. In those studies did anyone look at gastric emptying, because glucagon certainly inhibits gastric emptying. Somatostatin might do the same thing and the reduced xylose absorption may be purely an effect on gastric emptying.

Dr. Sperling
The problem with the gastric emptying studies is that they have been done at concentrations of glucagon which I do not think are physiological. The studies that have been done to inhibit gastric emptying used doses of glucagon in the order of one to two *milligrams*, as I recall, intravenously. That will raise glucagon concentrations to an astronomical range in terms of *picograms* per *ml*.. The normal concentration of glucagon which perfuses the portal circulation is of the order of 300-500 *picograms/ml*. I'm not sure whether that concentration is known to inhibit gastric emptying or gastric motility, but in radiological techniques people are now using large doses of glucagon, that is 1 - 2 *milligrams* intravenously, which are not physiological.

Dr. Ivey
You said that glucagon has been isolated in the A cells of the fundus of the stomach. Has anybody actually found it in the gastric juice?

Dr. Sperling
Well, there is no reason why it should be found in the gastric juice. If it is acting as a hormone or as a local hormone, it is either interacting with its neighboring cells or, being a hormone, it is by definition being secreted into the blood stream. Therefore, if it is in the gastric juice, it might be in very low concentrations, lesser concentrations than would be found in the blood stream.

Dr. Ivey
People have found gastrin in the gastric juice and feel like

it might have an important role there physiologically. I guess if it may be true of one hormone, then it may be true of others.

Dr. Sperling

But if you look at the gastrin-producing cells, particularly in patients with, say gastrinomas in the Zollinger-Ellison syndrome, they are far more numerous than are the glucagon-secreting cells. If you recall, what I said was that the glucagon-secreting cells in the fundus of the dog have been well characterized as true *alpha* cells with the electron microscopic, immunological, and biological characteristics of true pancreatic glucagon. In man, that has not yet been determined.

Dr. Gerich

I just returned from an international symposium on somatostatin, so I have some recent data that might pertain to Dr. Ivey's question.

Somatostatin has been found to be secreted into the gastric lumen and, presumably, then glucagon might also be. In terms of its effects on xylose absorption, of course no one has actually measured xylose absorption. They have looked at xylose appearance in blood after ingestion. A group in Stockholm has been looking at gastric transit time of glucose during the administration of somatostatin and find that this is markedly diminished. This suggests that some of the effect of somatostatin on blood xylose levels can be explained merely on the basis of transit time.

Naturally, our own studies where we feed patients three meals over a five-hour interval would suggest that abnormalities in absorption are not important. The patients have no gastrointestinal symptoms which would be expected with the consumption of large amounts of food over a five-hour period if its absorption had been inhibited.

In the studies where increased glucagon levels were noted with section of the umbilical cord, have you looked to see whether this might be mediated by adrenergic mechanisms?

Dr. Sperling

As pediatricians, we have been interested in the mechanisms which govern these adaptations in newborn life. The adaptations which one sees, the rise in glucagon, the fall in insulin, and the stabilization of blood glucose, and then the rise in free fatty acids and ketone bodies would be classical for an adrenergic mechanism. It suggests, at least superficially, that these effects might be mediated by epinephrine and, if that were the case, we ought to be able to mimic all, or many, of the neonatal events by infusing epinephrine or other adrenergic agonists with or without their respective *alpha* or *beta* blockers in utero. Obviously to do such experiments, one needs an animal model. One can't do that in human beings. This is why it was so crucially important for us to demonstrate that these changes also occur in the newborn lamb. So we've done these experiments and, as you will predict, the infusion of epinephrine to the fetus mimics all of the effects that I have described for you. We can show a rise in glucagon, a fall in insulin, and a rise in glucose.

Dr. Gerich

The conflicting opinions on glucagon that you have cited, based on my data and Dr. Felig's data, may be a little more exaggerated than people realize. We basically are finding the same things. Our group interprets them in one way and Dr. Felig interprets them in another way.

If you remember the slide showing the prolonged infusion of somatostatin for 18 hours in diabetes after we withdrew insulin, hyperglycemia definitely occurred to a level of about 150 *mg/dℓ*. So we don't believe that hyperglucagonemia is essential for the development of hyperglycemia but that in its absence the hyperglycemia is markedly attenuated.

I think the studies shown from Dr. Felig's work indicated the same thing. If you remember, when somatostatin was infused for about six hours, hyperglycemia resulted. But this was of a level of only 135 *mg/dℓ*. Now, since those studies were done in normal individuals, there was no way to produce just pure insulin deficiency. But a model for that is the pancreatectomized diabetic and recent studies from the group in England have shown that pancreatectomy is very similar to a somatostatin infusion. After withdrawal of insulin from pancreatectomized individuals who have been maintained normoglycemic by an infusion of insulin, blood ketone and glucose levels do not rise as much as in "regular" juvenile onset diabetics who have glucagon secretion.

So really the results of the three groups--the British group, my own, and Dr. Felig's--are very similar. We do not believe glucagon is essential for the metabolic consequences of insulin deficiency but that it can magnify these consequences.

Dr. Sperling

I tried very hard to give credit to that and say that it isn't the "essentiality" of the concept. I think the criticism is not to your studies but to another group of glucagon investigators who, in very reputable journals, propose the theory that glucagon is <u>essential</u> for the development of the metabolic abnormalities. So <u>what is</u> in question is the "essentiality" of glucagon for the development of the metabolic abnormalities. This I tried to stress.

I equally tried to stress that, without question, glucagon accelerates the rate of appearance of the metabolic abnormalities but it is not *per se* responsible for these metabolic abnormalities. The pancreatectomized model is an excellent one. When you look at those patients, their insulin requirements are about two-thirds those of usual juvenile diabetics and the rate of appearance of diabetic ketoacidosis following withdrawal is slower.

Incidentally, there is an analogous situation for pediatricians, which we have also worked on, and that is in the child with cystic fibrosis of the pancreas in whom destruction of insulin-secreting cells goes along with destruction of the glucagon-secreting *alpha* cells. Those of you who work with patients with cystic fibrosis know that when these patients develop diabetes, it is of a milder nature, and when they require insulin they usually require somewhere in the order of 15 to 20 units of insulin a day and rarely need 50 units. Moreover, they rarely develop ketoacidosis and when they do, the rate of development seems to be much, much lower than in the "brittle" type that we seen in the juvenile diabetic.

Dr. Burns

I regret that Dr. Unger isn't here to defend the "essentiality" concept. I find that, when I talk to proponents of these theories, my point-of-view reflects the point-of-view of the last one I talked to because they are always so persuasive and articulate that I come away convinced.

Dr. Haibach

You showed an impressive list of compounds that affect glucagon secretion. Are these the effects of physiological or pharmacological doses? If they are the effect of physiological doses, it would appear to be a jungle that is almost impossible to unravel.

Dr. Sperling

Not all the compounds that I listed were in physiological concentrations. For example, what are normal physiological concentrations of prostaglandins? One has no idea what the normal concentrations of prostaglandins are. One knows that if one takes an isolated perfused pancreas and perfuses it with prostaglandins that one can see a rise in glucagon before any change in insulin secretion. This is the work of Dr. Sumer Pek. The question therefore is, is this a physiological or pharmacological effect? That I cannot answer.

With some of the other hormones, for example, growth hormone, it probably is a physiological effect. We know that growth hormone profoundly affects development of the *beta* cells. In the absence of growth hormone, the ability to synthesize and secrete insulin is markedly attenuated. You can show this in growth hormone-deficient children. You can show that growth hormone-deficient children have a diabetic glucose tolerance test at a time when they have growth hormone deficiency because they have very poor insulin responses. If you treat these patients with growth hormone and allow the *beta* cells to grow, you find now a restoration of normal glucose tolerance and a restoration of normal insulin secretion with physiological doses of growth hormone.

Similarly, we have been able to show that in growth hormone-deficient children there is obtunded glucagon secretion. It isn't totally absent, but it is low when you compare it with the same children after a six-month period of growth hormone therapy. With samples always run in the same assay to avoid interassay variability, the same child consistently has greater glucagon responses to any kind of stimulus that we have tried after growth hormone therapy than before therapy.

So, many of these things probably are physiological. Certainly the calcium concentrations are probably physiological. But even if they are not physiological, they give us insights. And the "jungle," I think, equally applies to any other kind of hormone that one wants to study under normal circumstances. This is why investigators go to models such as the isolated islets of Langerhans, or the perfused rat pancreas, or what we did, which is to go to the blood-perfused dog pancreas to give us an insight as to what actually happens at physiological concentrations.

Dr. Werner

The effects that you showed with chronic somatostatin infusion were very interesting. With the variables that you mentioned, where the blood levels of insulin and glucagon change, one wonders what is really happening at the cell membranes and the receptors. We know that with hypoinsulinemia, certainly the receptors on the cells are increased, shifting the dose-response curve of insulin to the left so that smaller levels of insulin would give a better response. Could the data similarly be explained in that with hypoglucagonemia glucagon receptors might be even more increased on the cells so that the glucagon effect would persist?

So one asks, what would somatostatin do by changing hormonal blood levels and, second, what might somatostatin itself do to hormone receptors?

Dr. Sperling

I can't answer to the effects of somatostatin *per se* on hormone receptors. If Dr. Bar has data on that, I wish he would comment.

As far as the possibility that what we're seeing is that by lowering blood glucagon levels we raise the concentration or the affinity of the glucagon receptor on liver plasma cell membranes and, thereby, make the cell more responsive to the small doses of glucagon that prevail, that is very unlikely. It is unlikely because I don't think that the receptors change within a period of four to six hours. I think this is too rapid for the change to be seen. But it also is unlikely because with the glucagon receptor, I'm not sure that the same negative correlation exists as it does for the insulin receptor. As you pointed out, with hyperinsulinemia there is a decrease in the number of receptors. With hypoinsulinemia there is a rapid restoration of the number of insulin receptors. That may not be true for glucagon. For example, if you look at patients with chronic renal failure, they have hyperglucagonemia and they have an increased incidence of abnormal glucose tolerance. If you mimic this model in the rat and cause chronic renal failure, you will find again hyperglucagonemia but, despite the hyperglucagonemia, you find an increased sensitivity to generate cyclic AMP in a dose-response manner to increasing doses of glucagon. And in these animals when you look at the liver plasma cell membranes for glucagon, surprisingly and totally opposite to what has been seen in insulin, the number of binding sites for glucagon in the liver plasma cell membranes is increased in uremic rats and the amount of cyclic AMP generated in response to a small dose of glucagon is also increased, suggesting that it isn't just nonspecific binding, that it is actually an increase in the number of receptors. So the story of the glucagon receptor *vis-a-vis* the insulin receptor may not be the same and I don't think it explains these phenomena.

Dr. Werner

My question also related to the timing of effects; not going for days--

Dr. Sperling

You don't have to infuse somatostatin for days. You just have to infuse for four to six hours. After about two to three hours of low insulin and low glucagon, blood glucose rises. I think what happens, my own feeling without any data, is that the enzymatic machinery for insulin persists longer than that for glucagon after withdrawal of both insulin and glucagon. So that what may happen is that, as you acutely withdraw glucagon and insulin, the acute effects are those of the glucagon deficiency, with enzymatic machinery turned on by insulin persisting longer. Then, as the effects of insulin deficiency become predominant, you now see a rise in the glucose that takes two to three hours. I don't think that two to three hours would be soon enough to cause a change in receptors.

Dr. Brownlee

I was interested in your slide demonstrating that in the juvenile onset diabetic patients you were able to achieve normal suppression of glucagon by hyperglycemia in the presence of adequate insulin. Several years ago, unless I am not remembering correctly, Dr. Gerich demonstrated that there was also a blunted response to hypoglycemia in the stimulation of glucagon, while the response to arginine and other stimuli was apparently normal. This in conjunction with the nonsuppressibility by hyperglycemia, was taken as evidence of a specific glucoreceptor defect in the *alpha* cell. I wonder if you could comment on those two aspects in the light of your present data which suggests that one can normalize glucagon secretion with proper insulinization.

Dr. Sperling

As far as suppression is concerned, I don't think there is any question from all our studies--Dr. Gerich's studies now and Dr. Raskins' studies--that adequate therapy, in terms of normalization of metabolic abnormalities, through prolonged infusion of insulin or through strict control of the metabolic conditions will normalize the suppressive effects of glucose upon glucagon secretion.

Now, then, the question comes, what about the opposite end of the scale? The same holds true for the hyperresponsiveness to arginine. A strict period of metabolic control will normalize the hyperglucagonemic response to arginine. Nobody has found hyperglucagonemia in a prediabetic subjects. In prediabetic Pima Indians, for example, until they develop diabetes and relative insulin deficiency, there is no hyperresponsiveness of glucagon.

Let's go back to the opposite: You recall some of the data that Dr. Rubenstein presented yesterday. He pointed out that a Japanese group have now shown that the brittle diabetic, the one who has periods of hypoglycemia as well as hyperglycemia, has little C-peptide. These patients also have less response in terms of the glucagon rise during hypoglycemia.

I don't think anyone has yet done a period of strict control for two or three days with a chronic insulin infusion and then caused insulin-induced hypoglycemia to see whether that now allows them to find a normal acute response. Hyperglycemic suppression has been shown but acute hypoglycemia induced in juvenile diabetics does not cause an appropriate rise in glucagon.

Dr. Gerich

There is no question that the *alpha* cell is regulated by insulin secretion. If one infuses as little as one unit an hour to a juvenile diabetic, one can normalize the diabetic's response to arginine. This occurs over a matter of two to four hours. During that same time interval, we looked to see whether the diabetic *alpha* cells' abnormal suppressibility to hyperglycemia could be corrected by insulin, and we found that it could not. We have done 16-hour insulin infusions at a rate of one unit per hour. And we could not correct the diabetic *alpha* cell response to hypoglycemia.

The other studies of Raskin and our own studies have shown that we could get suppression of glucagon secretion to hyperglycemia by giving insulin, but the amount of insulin required was pharmacologic. No one has done the study you mentioned such as could be done by putting the patient on a Biostator, normalizing glucose homeostasis for a while, and then repeating the suppression. But the data to date suggest that the diabetic *alpha* cells respond differently to glucose than to arginine. You can correct the latter with small doses of insulin over a rapid period of time; the former you cannot.

So I think the concept of an abnormal glucose receptor is still a viable one and the extent to which it may depend on insulin secretion is the critical factor here.

SOMATOSTATIN--ANOTHER PANCREATIC ISLET HORMONE

John E. Gerich

Diabetes and Metabolism Research Laboratory
Departments of Medicine and Physiology
Mayo Medical School and Mayo Clinic
Rochester, MN 55901

INTRODUCTION

Pancreatic islets contain at least six different types of endocrine cells (Table 1). In most species A, B, and D cells comprise more than 75% of the islet cell mass. A and B cells secrete glucagon and insulin, respectively, and their role in substrate homeostasis is well established. Although D cells were first described shortly after the discovery of A and B cells (Bensley, 1911), much less is known about them and their function. Initially, the D cell was thought to be merely an intermediary

*Table 1. ENDOCRINE CELLS OF MAMMALIAN ISLETS OF LANGERHANS**

Cell type	Secretory product	Percent islet cell mass
B	Insulin	40-60
A	Glucagon	20-30
D	Somatostatin	5-15
F	Pancreatic polypeptide	5-15
D_1	Vasoactive intestinal peptide	0-5
EC	Serotonin	0-5

**Modified from Revised Wiesbaden Classification: Rendic. Gastroenterol. (1973) 5:13-16.*

Table 2. STAINING CHARACTERISTICS OF PANCREATIC A, B, AND D CELLS

Stain	A cell	B cell	D cell
Chrome-hematoxylin-phloxin	pink	dark blue	pink
Phosphotungstic acid hematoxylin	dark grey	unstained	pale lilac
Heidenhains azan	red	pale	blue
Aldehyde fuchsin-trichome	red	violet	green
Silver impregnation (Hellman-Hellerstrom)	yellow	yellow	black
Fluorescein-labeled antisera:			
a. antiglucagon	+	-	-
b. antiinsulin	-	+	-
c. antisomatostatin	-	-	+

form of A cell due to the poor resolution of A and D cells with stains used to study islet morphology and to the fact that argyrophilic islet cells were mistakenly considered A cells (Takahashi, 1927). With the introduction of improved staining techniques (azan staining and the counterstaining of aldehyde-fuschin sections by the trichome method, Table 2), the D cell became recognized as a distinct entity (for review see Fujita, 1968). Indeed, as early as 1937 Thomas reported, in a comprehensive morphologic study (Thomas, 1937), the presence of D cells in all mammalian islets he examined. Some time later, doubt arose as to identity of the argyrophil and A cell, since not all phloxin-positive (A) cells were argyrophilic. This led to a subdivision of A cells into A_1 (phloxin-positive, silver-positive) and A_2 (phloxin-positive, silver-negative) cells (Hellman, Wallgren, and Hellerstrom, 1962). By 1964 it was established that the A_1 cell was the D cell, and the A_2 became simply the A cell (Fujita, 1964). Although changes in D cell morphology had been described in various pathologic conditions (Fujita, 1968), little was known of its possible function until recently when several laboratories established that it contained somatostatin (Dubois, 1975; Hokfelt, Effendic, Hellerstrom, Johansson, Luft, and Arimura, 1975; Orci, Baetens, and Rufener, 1975; Polak, Grimelius, Pearse, Bloom, and Arimura, 1975). The purpose of this paper is to review the present state of knowledge concerning pancreatic D cell function.

BACKGROUND

Somatostatin, the secretory product of D. cells, is a tetradecapeptide (Figure 1), which was originally isolated from the hypo-

H-ALA-GLY-CYS-LYS-ASN-PHE-PHE-TRP-LYS-THR-PHE-THR-SER-CYS-OH

Figure 1. Primary sequence of somatostatin

Table 3. SUMMARY OF REPORTED BIOLOGIC ACTIONS OF SOMATOSTATIN

Endocrine: (inhibits secretion of)	Nonendocrine: (diminishes or prevents)
growth hormone	gastric emptying, HCl and pepsin secretion
thyrotropin	pancreatic bicarbonate and enzyme release
prolactin+,++	gallbladder contraction
ACTH++	xylose and triglyceride absorption
insulin	splanchnic blood flow*
pancreatic and gut glucagon	platelet aggregation**
gastric inhibitory polypeptide	LD_{50} Phenobarbital
vasoactive intestinal peptide	CNS neuronal electrical activity
secretin	myenteric plexus acetylcholine release
pancreozymin	
gastrin	
motilin	
pancreatic polypeptide	
renin	

+not all species
++not in normal tissue

*may not be direct effect
**disputed

thalamus (Burgus, Ling, Butcher, and Guillemin, 1973). Because of its ability to inhibit growth hormone secretion, it was considered at that time to be a hypothalamic factor. Subsequently, among other actions (Table 3), somatostatin was discovered to be a potent inhibitor of insulin and glucagon secretion (for review see Gerich, 1976). Then, using antiserum generated against synthetic somatostatin, it was soon found by immunohistochemical means (*vide supra*) and by radioimmunoassay (Arimura, Sato, Dupont, Nishi, and Schally, 1975; Patel and Weir, 1976) that pancreatic islets of various spe-

Table 4. SPECIES WHOSE PANCREAS CONTAINS SOMATOSTATIN

Catfish	Hagfish	Pig
Chicken	Horse	Pigeon
Chinese Hamster	Man	Rat
Frog	Mouse	Sheep
Guinea Pig	Ox	Torpedo

cies contained a substance immunologically similar to somatostatin (Table 4). Since most of this immunoreactivity coelutes with synthetic somatostatin on gel chromatography and inhibits growth hormone release from cultured pituitary cells in parallel with the native and synthetic molecules (Vale, Brazeau, Rivier, Brown, Bass, Burgus, Ling, and Guillemin, 1975; Vale, Ling, Rivier, Villarreal, Rivier, Brown, and Douglas, 1976), its identity with somatostatin is now generally accepted. Moreover, the ability of isolated islets to synthesize somatostatin *in vitro* has recently been demonstrated (Ensinck, Laschansky, Kanter, Fujimoto, Koerker, and Goodner, 1978; Noe, Weir, and Bauer, 1978). This indicates that the somatostatin present in islets *in vivo* is not merely the result of its being taken up from other sources (*e.g.*, circulation, nerve endings).

The ability of somatostatin to inhibit insulin and glucagon secretion and its presence within islets suggests that it may function as a regulator of the secretion of these hormones and, also, in view of the importance of insulin and glucagon in substrate homeostasis, that somatostatin may indirectly act as a modulator of nutrient flux. Major questions, at the present time, are:

> Under what circumstances does somatostatin affect insulin and glucagon release?
>
> Does it affect the release of each hormone equally or preferentially?
>
> Are there separate populations of D cells (one for A cells and one for B cells)?
>
> How is D cell function related to abnormalities of A and B cell function?

While most of these questions remain unanswered, some insight into D cell function has come about mainly from four sources: correlative studies of A, B, and D cell morphology; studies of somatostatin secretion; studies utilizing somatostatin antiserum to neutralize the effects of endogenous somatostatin; and examination of the effects of excessive secretion of somatostatin by pancreatic D cell tumors.

MORPHOLOGIC STUDIES

In most mammalian species, D cells resemble A cells in size, being somewhat smaller than B cells. Their shape is highly variable, crescent, spindle, oval, and polygonal forms having been described (Fujita, 1968). Most characteristic of the D cell are its cytoplasmic granules as seen in electronmicrographs (Figure 2). In contrast to A and B cells, granules of the D cell contain no halo; their electron density is intermediate between the paler B and darker A cell granules, and their size appears to vary more than those of A and B cells.

The content and distribution of somatostatin in pancreatic islets varies widely among species (Fujita, 1968; Vale *et al.*, 1976) and, indeed, even among different areas of the same species (Weir, Goltsos, Steinberg, and Patel, 1976). Pancreases of fowl such as the pigeon and chicken have the highest content of somatostatin. In these species, whose pancreas contains three types of islets (light, dark, and mixed), D cells are situated in association with B cells in light islets and with A cells in dark islets (Fujita, 1968). In the rat (Orci and Unger, 1975) and horse (Helmstaedter, Feurle, and Forssmann, 1976), D cells occupy the periphery of islets associated with A cells in the former species and with B cells in the latter. In man (Figure 3) and the guinea pig (Dubois, 1975; Hokfelt *et al.*, 1975), D cells are randomly scattered throughout islets, as are A and B cells. Thus, no generalized anatomic relationship exists between D cells and either A or B cells in all species and caution must be exercised in extrapolating findings in one species to functional relationship in others.

Early studies of D cell ontogenesis suggest that it may precede the development of A and B cells in some species (see Fujita 1968 for review) but these investigations antedate immunologic techniques and precise definition of islet cell types. Immunoreactive somatostatin has been identified in the human fetal pan-

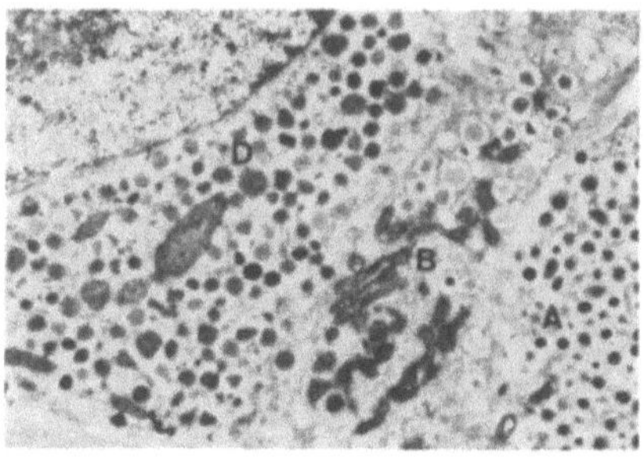

Figure 2. Electronmicrograph of rat pancreatic islet. D = D cell, B = B cell, A = A cell (courtesy of Dr. Lelio Orci).

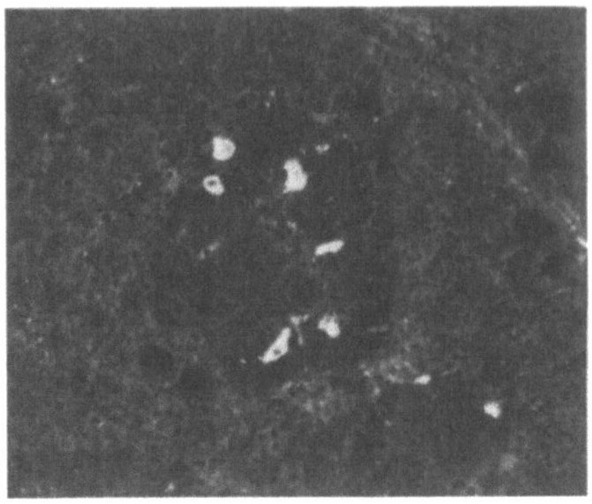

Figure 3. Human pancreatic islet stained by indirect fluorescence technique against somatostatin (courtesy of Dr. Lelio Orci).

creas (Dubois, Paulin, Assan, and Dubois, 1975). Changes in D cell number or pancreatic somatostatin content have been observed under a variety of conditions. Several workers, using conventional microscopy, noted increased numbers of argyrophilic or A_1 cells in pancreases from diabetic humans (Creutzfeldt, 1956; Ferner, 1942, Fujita, 1966; Gepts, 1958) and alloxan diabetic rats (Hellman and Petersson, 1963; Kobayashi, Takahashi, and Johshita, 1964). These most likely represented changes in D cells since Orci and his colleagues (Orci, Baetens, Rufner, Amherdt, Ravazzola, Studer, Malaisse-Lagae, and Unger, 1976), using immunofluorescent techniques, have recently reported hyperplasia of D cells in pancreases of rats made diabetic with alloxan and in pancreases of humans with juvenile-onset type diabetes (Figure 4); and others (Makino, Kanatsuka, Matsushima, Yamamoto, Kumagai, and Yanaihara, 1977; Patel and Weir, 1976) found increased immunoreactive somatostatin in pancreases of rats made diabetic with streptozotocin. However, diminished pancreatic somatostatin has been reported (Patel, Orci, Bankier, and Cameron, 1976) in two strains of obese spontaneously diabetic mice (db/db and ob/ob). These animals, in contrast to those with induced diabetes, are hyperinsulinemic. Increased numbers of D cells have been reported in association with nonD-cell islet tumors (insulinomas, gastrinomas, VIPomas) and in nesidioblastosis (Bloom, Polak, and West, 1978; Heitz, Kloppel, Hacki, Polak, and Pearse, 1977). Whether these alterations are part of the basic pathologic process or are merely compensatory changes remains to be established.

SOMATOSTATIN SECRETION

Somatostatin secretion *in vitro* from incubated rat islets or from perfused canine pancreases has been examined in several labor-

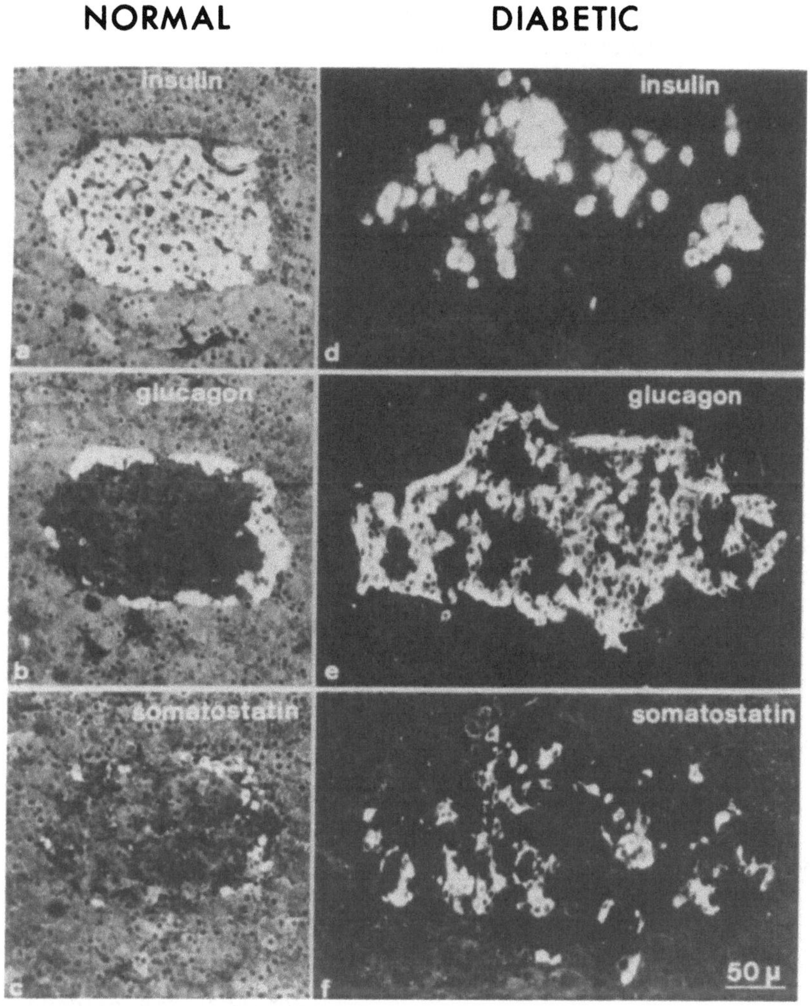

Figure 4. Serial sections of pancreatic islet from normal (a,b,c) and alloxan diabetic (d.e.f) rats stained with fluorescein-labeled antiserum against insulin (a,d), glucagon (b,e), and somatostatin (c,f) (courtesy Dr. Lelio Orci).

atories. The results of these studies are summarized in Table 5. Somatostatin release is stimulated by glucose (Ipp, Patton, Dobbs, Harris, Vale, and Unger, 1977; Schauder, McIntosh, Arends, Arnold, Frerichs, and Creutzfeldt, 1976, 1977; Weir, Samols, Ramseur, Day, and Patel, 1977), arginine (Patton, Ipp, Dobbs, Orci, Vale, and Unger, 1976), leucine (Schauder *et al.*, 1977), glucagon (Patton *et al.*, 1977), isoproterenol (Samols, Weir, Patel, Loo, and Gabbay, 1977), gut hormones (Ipp, Harris, Dobbs, Arimura, Vale, and Unger, 1977), and substances which elevate islet cAMP levels such as theophylline and 8-BR-cAMP (Barden, Alvarado-Urbina, Cote, and Dupont,

Table 5. SUMMARY OF FACTORS AFFECTING SECRETION OF SOMATOSTATIN BY PANCREATIC D CELLS

Agent	Effect on somatostatin release
Substrates	
glucose	stimulation
arginine	stimulation
leucine	stimulation
ketoisocaproic acid	stimulation
glyceraldehyde	inhibition
Hormones	
glucagon	stimulation
insulin	no effect
epinephrine	inhibition
acetylcholine	inhibition
GIP	stimulation
gastrin	stimulation
pancreozymin	stimulation
secretin	stimulation
Miscellaneous	
theophylline	stimulation
8-BR-cAMP	stimulation
isoproterenol	stimulation
mannoheptulose	inhibition
antimycin	inhibition
diazoxide	inhibition

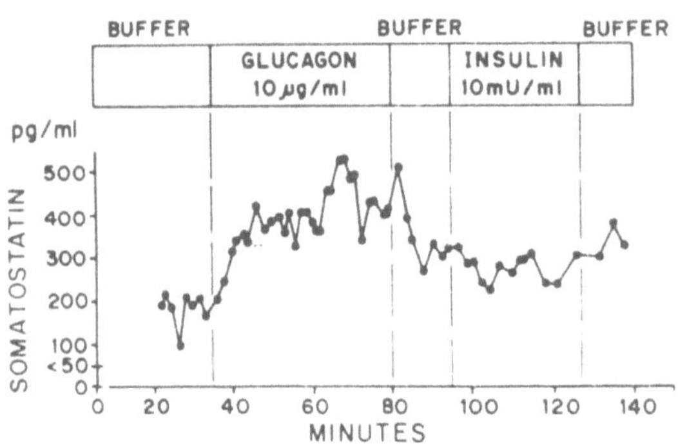

Figure 5. Effect of exogenous glucagon and insulin on somatostatin release from canine pancreas perfused in vitro (courtesy Dr. Gloria Patton).

1976; Schauder *et al.*, 1977), whereas epinephrine (Shauder *et al.*, 1976), acetylcholine (Samols *et al.*, 1977), and inhibitors of cellular metabolism (Schauder *et al.*, 1976) decrease somatostatin release. The effect of glucagon and insulin infusions on somatostatin secretion is shown in Figure 5. Thus, D cell function may be under metabolic, normonal, and neural (autonomic) control as are A and B cell function (Gerich and Lorenzi, 1977).

Most agents which increase somatostatin release also increase insulin release. Since insulin itself does not appear to acutely affect somatostatin release (Patton *et al.*, 1977), these agents most likely exert their effects directly on the D cell. Whether the somatostatin released under these conditions affects insulin secretion is unclear, since one would expect an inverse relationship between insulin and somatostatin release; however, one might argue that insulin responses would be greater if somatostatin were not secreted. At the present time a more plausible argument can be made for somatostatin control of glucagon release. Stimulation of somatostatin release by glucagon could be part of a negative feedback system and could also explain the ability of arginine, a potent glucagon secretagogue, to stimulate somatostatin release. Suppression of glucagon secretion by glucose might be mediated through the augmentation of somatostatin release by glucose. Moreover, the suppression of somatostatin release by mannoheptulose, epinephrine, and acetylcholine could be responsible for the increase in glucagon secretion occurring with these agents (Gerich, Charles, and Grodsky, 1976). However, with this rather simple and, perhaps, naïve relationship between A and D cell function, one has difficulty explaining how agents such as the various gut hormones and isoproterenol augment release of both somatostatin and glucagon unless one postulates that these agents affect somatostatin release indirectly through their effect on glucagon secretion.

Although immunoreactive somatostatin-like substances have been detected in the general circulation (Pimstone, Kronheim, and Berelowitz, 1977), there is controversy whether these truly represent authentic tetradecapeptide and, if so, what their origin is (hypothalamus, thyroid, gut, pancreas). Suffice it to say that data, at this time, is quite limited. Nevertheless, "elevated" circulating levels of immunoreactive somatostatin have been found in patients wiht pancreatic D cell tumors (Larsson, Holst, Kuhl, Hirsch, Ingemansson, Jensen, Rehfeld, and Schwartz, 1977) and in dogs made diabetic with alloxan (Unger and Orci, 1978).

STUDIES WITH SOMATOSTATIN ANTISERUM

Intraperitoneal administration of antiserum against somatostatin augments growth hormone and thyrotropin secretion but has no effect on plasma levels of glucose, insulin, and glucagon (Arimura and Schally, 1976; Arimura, Smith, and Schally, 1976; Stewart, Steiner, Barber, Koerker, Goodner, and Gale, 1977). These results support a role for circulating somatostatin (hypothalamic-pituitary portal system) as a physiologic regulator of growth hormone and thyrotropin secretion but not of insulin and glucagon secretion. Conceivably antiserum so administered may not have had access to somatostatin released by D cells into the islet microvasculature. In two recent studies, release of insulin alone and both insulin and glucagon from isolated rat islets incubated with antiserum against somatostatin have been examined. In one study (Barden *et al.*, 1977), no effect on insulin release was observed while marked augmentation of glucagon release occurred (Figure 6); in the other study (Taniguchi, Utsumi, Hasegawa, Kobayashi, Watanabe, Murakami, Seki, Tsutou, Makimura, Sakoda, and Baba, 1977), insulin release at glucose concentrations below 9 mM was augmented while no effect of the antiserum was observed at 16.7 mM glucose concentration. Since both studies used comparable glucose levels, the reason for the conflicting data on insulin release is unclear. Nevertheless, taken together these reports provide evidence for a regulatory role of locally released (paracrine) somatostatin on adjacent islet cell function.

SOMATOSTATINOMAS

To date, two well documented cases of pancreatic D cell tumors secreting somatostatin have been reported. In one case (Ganda, Weir, Soeldner, Legg, Chick, Patel, Ebeid, Gabbay, and Reichlin, 1977) the tumor was benign and released immunoreactive somatostatin in tissue culture. In the other case (Larsson *et al.*, 1977) the tumor was malignant, its venous effluent had markedly elevated im-

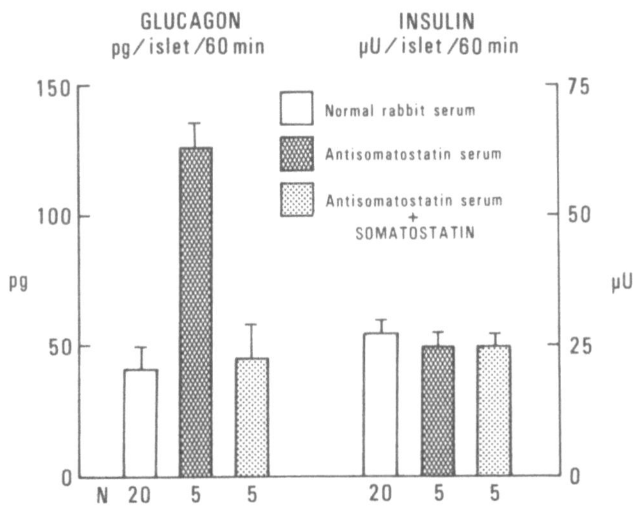

Figure 6. Effect of antisomatostatin serum on glucagon and insulin release from isolated rat islets incubated in vitro (data from Barden et al., 1977).

munoreactive somatostatin, and extracts of the tumor coeluted with synthetic somatostatin on gel chromatography and inhibited secretion of insulin and glucagon *in vitro*. The clinical features of both cases had interesting similarities. In each instance the patient had mild diabetes despite markedly impoverished insulin release. Presumably, this attenuation of diabetes was the result of the combined inhibition of glucagon and insulin secretion by the tumor somatostatin (Gerich, 1977). Removal of the benign tumor led to complete remission of diabetes. These reports clearly indicate that endogenous somatostatin can, under certain circumstances, influence pancreatic A and B cell function sufficiently to alter glucose homeostasis. Whether pancreatic somatostatin affects gastrointestinal function is unclear, since one patient had normal gastric acid secretion and no evidence of disturbed gastrointestinal or pancreatic exocrine function whereas the other patient had signs of malabsorption. However, the latter patient had a large malignant tumor which could have caused these effects by extension into adjacent tissues rather than by release of somatostatin.

SUMMARY AND CONCLUSION

While it is firmly established that somatostatin is another islet hormone, its function and its relationship to insulin and glucagon are still unclear. Studies to date have not yet provided conclusive evidence that somatostatin regulates A or B cell function, although such a role seems likely. It has been suggested (Unger, Ipp, Schusdziarra, and Orci, 1977) that somatostatin may be part of a "gut-islet-gut" axis in which gastrointestinal hormones stimulate somatostatin secretion, which then inhibits gastrointestinal activities to provide more coordinated entry of exogenous nutrients. That endogenous somatostatin can alter carbohydrate homeostasis seems clear from the clinical picture in patients with somatostatin-secreting islet D cell tumors. Although insulin, in contrast to glucagon, does not seem to affect somatostatin secretion acutely, prolonged excess or deficiency of insulin may alter D cell function. The intriguing discovery of alterations in islet D cell mass and somatostatin content in insulinopenic and insulinoplethoric diabetes in man and experimental animals raises the possibility that abnormal D cell function may contribute to some of the metabolic disturbances observed in these forms of diabetes. It can be concluded with reasonable confidence that, over the next few years, studies of islet D cell function will surely continue to enhance our understanding of nutrient homeostasis.

REFERENCES

Arimura, A., Sato, H., Dupont, A., Nishi, N., and Schally, A. 1975. Somatostatin: Abundance of immunoreactive hormone in rat stomach and pancreas. *Science* 189:1007-1008.

Arimura, A. and Schally, A. 1976. Increase in basal and thyrotropin-releasing hormone (TRH)-stimulated secretion of thyrotropin (TSH) by passive immunization with antiserum to somatostatin in rats. *Endocrinology* **98**:1069-1072.

Arimura, A., Smith, W., and Schally, A. 1976. Blockage of the stress-induced decrease in blood GH by anti-somatostatin serum in rats. *Endocrinology* **98**:540-543.

Barden, N., Lavoie, M., Dupont, A., Cote, J., and Cote, J-P. 1977. Stimulation of glucagon release by addition of antisomatostatin serum to islets of Langerhans *in vitro*. *Endocrinology* **101**:635-637.

Bensley, R. 1911. Studies on the pancreas of the guinea pig. *Am. J. Anat.* **12**:297-388.

Bloom, S., Polak, J., and West, A. 1978. Somatostatin content of pancreatic endocrine tumors. *Metabolism* **27**:1235-1238.

Burgus, R., Ling, N., Butcher, M., and Guillemin, R. 1973. Primary structure of somatostatin, a hypothalamic peptide that inhibits the secretion of pituitary growth hormone. *Proc. Nat. Acad. Sci.* USA **70**:684-688.

Creutzfeldt, W. 1953. Zur deutung des silberzellbildes und anderer pankreasbefunde beim diabetes mellitus und inseladenom. *Beitrg. Pathol. Anat.* 113:133-168.

Dubois, M. 1975. Immunoreactive somatostatin is present in discrete cells of the endocrine pancreas. *Proc. Nat. Acad. Sci.* USA 72:1340-1343.

Dubois, P., Paulin, C., Assan, R., and Dubois, M. 1975. Evidence for immunoreactive somatostatin in the endocrine cells of human foetal pancreas. *Nature* **256**:731-732.

Ensinck, J., Laschansky, E., Kanter, R., Fujimoto, W., Koerker, D., and Goodner, C. 1978. Somatostatin biosynthesis and release in the hypothalamus and pancreas of the rat. *Metabolism* **27**:1207-1210.

Ferner, H. 1942. Beiträge zur histologie der Langerhansschen inseln des menschen mit besonderer berücksichtigung der silberzellen und ihrer beziehung zum pankreasdiabetes. *Virchows Arch. Pathol. Anat.* **309**:87-136.

Fujita, T. 1964. The identification of the argyrophil cells of pancreatic islets with D cells. *Arch. Histol. Jap.* **25**:189-197.

Fujita, T. 1966. D-zellen der pankreasinseln beim diabetes mellitus mit besonderer berücksichtigung ihrer argyrophilie. *Z. Zellforsch* **69**:363-370.

Fujita, T. 1968. D cell, the third endocrine element of the pancreatic islet. *Arch. Histol. Jap.* **29**:1-40.

Ganda, O., Weir, G., Soeldner, J., Legg, M., Chick, W., Patel, Y., Ebeid, A., Gabbay, K., and Reichlin, S. 1977. Somatostatinoma: A somatostatin containing tumor of the endocrine pancreas. *N. Eng. J. Med.* **296**:963-967.

Gepts, W. 1958. Die histopathologischen veranderungen des Langerhansschen inseln und ihrer bedeutung in der frage der pathogenese des menschlichen diabetes. *Endokrinologie* **36**:185-211.

Gerich, J.E. 1976. Somatostatin and the endocrine pancreas. IN F. Labrie, J. Meites, and G. Pelletier (Eds.) *Current topics in molecular endocrinology*. Vol. III. *Hypothalamus and endocrine functions*. New York: Plenum Press.

Gerich, J.E. 1977. Somatostatin--its possible role in carbohydrate homeostasis and the treatment of diabetes mellitus. *Arch. Int. Med.* 137:656-666.

Gerich, J., Charles, M., and Grodsky, G. 1976. Regulation of pancreatic insulin and glucagon secretion. *Ann. Rev. Physiol.* **38**:353-388.

Gerich, J. and Lorenzi, M. 1977. The role of the autonomic nervous system and somatostatin in the control of insulin and glucagon secretion. IN W. Ganong and L. Martini (Eds.) *Frontiers in neuroendocrinology*. Vol. 5. New York: Raven Press.

Heitz, P., Kloppel, G., Hacki, W., Polak, J., and Pearse, A. 1977. Nesidioblastosis: The pathologic basis of persistent hyperinsulinemic hypoglycemia in infants: Morphologic and quantitive analysis of seven cases based on specific immunostaining and electron microscopy. *Diabetes* **26**:632-642.

Hellman, B. and Petersson, G. 1963. Long term changes of the A_1 and A_2 cells in the islets of rats with alloxan diabetes. *Endocrinology* **72**:238-242.

Hellman, B., Wallgren, A., and Hellerstrom, C. 1962. Two types of islet A cells in different parts of the pancreas of the dog. *Nature* **194**:1201-1202.

Helmstaedter, V., Feurle, G., and Forssmann, W. 1976. Insulin-, glucagon-, and somatostatin-immunoreactive endocrine cells in the equine pancreas. *Cell Tiss. Res.* **172**:447-454.

Hokfelt, T., Effendic, S., Hellerstrom, C., Johansson, O., Luft, R., and Arimura, A. 1975. Cellular localization of somatostatin in endocrine-like cells and neurons of the rat with special references to the A_1-cells of the pancreatic islets and to the hypothalamus. *Acta Endocrinologica* **80**(Suppl. 200): 1-41.

Ipp, E., Dobbs, R., Harris, V., Arimura, A., VAle, W., and Unger, R. 1977. The effects of gastrin, GIP, secretin, and the octapeptide of cholecystokinin upon immunoreactive somatostatin release by the perfused canine pancreas. *J. Clin. Invest.* **60**: in press.

Ipp, E., Patton, G., Dobbs, R., Harris, V., Vale, W., and Unger, R. 1977. Endogenous immunoreactive somatostatin secretion by the pancreas. *Diabetes* **26**(Suppl. 1):359.

Kobayashi, K., Takahashi, Y., and Johshita, T. 1964. Influences of alloxan administration and hypophysectomy on the pancreatic islets of the rat. *Arch. Histol. Jap.* **25**:199-216.

Larsson, L., Holst, J., Kuhl, C., Hirsch, M., Ingemansson, S., Jensen, S., Rehfeld, J., and Schwartz, T. 1977. Pancreatic somatostatinoma: Clinical features and physiologic implications. *Lancet* **1**:666-668.

Makino, H., Kanatsuka, A., Matsushima, Y., Yamamoto, M., Kumagai, A., and Yanaihara, N. 1977. Effect of streptozotocin administration on somatostatin content of pancreas and hypothalamus in rats. *Endocrinol. Japon.* **24**:295-299.

Noe, B., Weir, G., and Bauer, G. 1978. Biosynthesis of somatostatin in pancreatic islets. *Metabolism* **27**:1201-1205.

Orci, L., Baetens, D., and Rufener, C. 1975. Evidence for the D-cell of the pancreas secreting somatostatin. *Horm. Metab. Res.* **7**:400-406.

Orci, L., Baetens, D., Rufener, C., Amherdt, M., Ravazzola, M., Studer, P., Malaisse-Lagae, F., and Unger, R. 1976. Hypertrophy and hyperplasia of somatostatin-containing D-cells in diabetes. *Proc. Nat. Acad. Sci.* USA **73**:1338-1342.

Orci, L. and Unger, R. 1975. Functional subdivision of islets of Langerhans and possible role of D cells. *Lancet* **2**:1243-1244.

Patel, Y., Orci, L., Bankier, A., and Cameron, D. 1976. Decreased pancreatic somatostatin (SRIF) concentration in spontaneously diabetic mice. *Endocrinology* **99**:1415-1418.

Patel, Y. and Weir, G. 1976. Increased somatostatin content of islets from streptozotocin-diabetic rats. *Clin. Endocrinol.* **5**:191-194.

Patton, G., Ipp, E., Dobbs, R., Orci, L., Vale, W., and Unger, R. 1976. Response of pancreatic immunoreactive somatostatin to arginine. *Life. Sci.* **19**:1957-1960.

Patton, G., Ipp, E., Dobbs, R., Orci, L., Vale, W., and Unger, R. 1977. Pancreatic immunoreactive somatostatin release. *Proc. Nat. Acad. Sci.* USA **74**:2140-2143.

Pimstone, B., Kronheim, S., and Berelowitz, M. 1977. The characterization of somatostatin-like immunoreactivity in human and rat serum. *Diabetes* **26**(Suppl. 1):359.

Polak, J., Grimelius, L., Pearse, A., Bloom, S., and Arimura, A. 1975. Growth-hormone release-inhibiting hormone in gastrointestinal and pancreatic D cells. *Lancet* **1**:1220-1222.

Samols, E., Weir, G., Patel, Y., Loo, S., and Gabbay, K. 1977. Autonomic control of somatostatin and pancreatic polypeptide secretion by the isolated perfused canine pancreas. *Clin. Res.* **25**:499A.

Schauder, P., McIntosh, C., Arends, J., Arnold, R., Frerichs, H., and Creutzfeldt, W. 1976. Somatostatin and insulin release from isolated rat pancreatic islets stimulated by glucose. *FEBS Lett.* **68**:225-227.

Solcia, E., Pearse, A., Grube, D., Kobayashi, S., Bussolate, G., Creutzfeldt, W., and Gepts, W. 1973. Revised Wiesbaden classification of gut endocrine cells. *Rendic. Gastroenterol.* **5**:13-16.

Stewart, J., Steiner, R., Barber, J., Koerker, D., Goodner, C., and Gale, C. 1977. Effects of active immunization against somatostatin on secretion of growth hormone and insulin in adolescent male baboons. *Endocrinology* **100**:230.

Takahashi, T. 1927. Uber die silberreaktion in den Langerhansschen inseln. *Trans. Jap. Pathol. Soc.* **17**:65-66.

Taniguchi, H., Utsumi, M., Hasegawa, M., Kogayashi, T., Watanabe, Y., Murakami, K., Seki, M., Tsutou, A., Makimura, H., Sakoda, M., and Baba, S. 1977. Physiologic role of somatostatin: Insulin release from rat islets treated with somatostatin antiserum. *Diabetes* **26**:700-702.

Thomas, T. 1937. Cellular components of the islets of Langerhans. *Am. J. Anat.* **62**:31-57.

Unger, R., Ipp, E., Schusdziarra, V., and Orci, L. 1977. Hypothesis: Physiologic role of pancreatic somatostatin and the contribution of D-cell disorders to diabetes mellitus. *Life Sci.* **20**:2081-2086.

Unger, R. and Orci, L. 1978. Pancreatic somatostatin, a regulator of nutrient homeostasis: Normal and diabetic secretory patterns. *Metabolism* (in press).

Vale, W., Brazeau, P., Rivier, C., Brown, M., Boss, B., Rivier, J., Burgus, R., Ling, N., and Guillemin, R. 1975. Somatostatin. *Rec. Prog. Horm. Res.* **34**:365-397.

Vale, W., Ling, N. Rivier, J., Villarreal, J., Rivier, C., Brown, M., and Douglas, C. 1976. Anatomic and phylogenetic distribution of somatostatin. *Metabolism* **25**(Suppl. 1):1491-1494.

Weir, G., Goltsos, P., Steinberg, E., and Patel, Y. 1976. High concentration of somatostatin immunoreactivity in chicken pancreas. *Diabetologia* **12**:129-132.

Weir, G., Samols, E., Ramseur, R., Day, J., and Patel, Y. 1977. Influence of glucose and glucagon upon somatostatin secretion from the isolated perfused canine pancreas. *Clin. Res.* **25**:403A.

DISCUSSION FOLLOWING DR. GERICH'S TALK

Dr. Burns

Thank you very much, Dr. Gerich, for a very clear presentation. You didn't mention, very much at least, the pervasive distribution of somatostatin throughout the central nervous system. I wonder if you would want to comment on its role as viewed from that perspective.

Dr. Gerich

In addition to being found in the islets of Langerhans and in the hypothalamus, somatostatin is in various other parts of the central nervous system and is also found in the stomach, duodenum, and ileum. In some studies where the hypothalamus is isolated surgically, it has been found that the somatostatin content of the "island" will almost totally disappear. This indicates that the somatostatin found in the hypothalamus is probably made elsewhere and secreted down nerve endings into the basal hypothalamus. Currently it is thought that these cell bodies may be present in the anterior part of the hypothalamus. Somatostatin has also been found in the spinal cord and in peripheral sensory ganglia.

So, currently, we have several potential roles of somatostatin: one, as a neurohormone-regulating pituitary function as a local regulator of insulin and glucagon secretion and of gastrointestinal function and, lastly, as a possible neurotransmitter--both in the peripheral and central nervous system. Somatostatin has also been found in gastric secretions. So it is quite conceivable that locally released somatostatin may spill over and have a function on adjacent gastric cells.

Dr. Sperling

Two questions: One, the initial work of John Ensink suggested it was impossible to measure somatostatin in biological fluids. In line with that, people who have tried to measure LRH or TRH have been rather unsuccessful, whereas the more recent reports suggest that, in fact, they can be measured in bological fluids.

I wonder if you might comment on the differences and what this means?

Secondly, could you answer whether there have been measurements of somatostatin in biological fluids, in plasma in diabetic animal models, or in humans rather than the studies that you showed which were essentially in isolated islets?

Dr. Gerich

Well, in answer to your first question, there is considerable controversy about immunoreactive somatostatin in the peripheral circulation. Part of this may be due to different antiserums that are used and partly due to interfering factors in plasma. There are now four groups who claim to measure somatostatin in the circulation. One group uses EDTA to prevent proteolysis. Some claim that extraction is necessary. The studies of Pimstone have been the most exhaustive in trying to show that what is picked up as immunoreactive somatostatin is identical to the tetradecapeptide. He has done column chromatography and found that it coelutes with synthetic somatostatin.

I know, however, of no biologic data where they have taken plasma, put it over a column, lyophilized it, and then checked to see whether it will prevent growth hormone secretion. The only such studies are from portal venous blood in the patient with the somatostatinoma.

In regard to your second question about altered somatostatin secretion in perhaps an animal model of diabetes, I have heard that Pimstone looked at this in alloxan-treated animals and found higher levels in the portal vein but not peripherally. At a recent meeting Roger Unger reported increased portal and peripheral levels. It's known that in many studies one can get very large changes of glucagon in the portal circulation but none, let's say, in the femoral artery. So we may also be dealing with the question of the sensitivity of the systems.

Dr. Haibach

Somatostatin has been shown to change the blood flow in the splanchnic system and affect peptide hormone secretion there. In addition, I think it has been shown to change the flow in the pituitary portan system and change peptide synthesis there as well.

Has peptide hormone synthesis in the parathyroid gland and in the parafollicular cells of the thyroid been studied in this regard?

Dr. Gerich

In terms of the splanchnic blood flow, several groups have found that it decreases splanchnic blood flow.

Somatostatin is found in the parafollicular cells. It does not affect calcitonin or parathyroid hormone secretion. But recently, it has been found to diminish T-3 secretion from human thyroid *in vitro*, and, when infused into normal humans, to diminish the rise in T-3 that occurs after TSH secretion.

Now, there seems to be a parallel between where somatostatin is found and a biologic action. There is only one exception to this; this is its effect on renin secretion. It lowers renin secretion but has not yet been found in the kidney. This may just be a sensitivity problem of the assays.

Dr. Levine

I want to get back to that question having to do with xylose absorption. Has anybody studied the effect of somatostatin on absorption *in vitro* of glucose and xylose, and some of the other nonmetabolizing sugars?

Dr. Gerich

Yes. A small effect was observed.

Dr. Weinstein

You mentioned the widespread distribution of somatostatin in the nervous system. We know that transport of glucose in nervous tissue does not respond to insulin.

In regard to glucose metabolism, do you have any evidence or can you postulate perhaps the metabolic role of somatostatin in the nervous system?

Dr. Gerich

Well, to date virtually all studies of the effect of somatostatin on glucose production or utilization have indicated that it does not, itself, have a direct effect. There are some elegant studies that appeared in *Diabetes* looking at the effects of somatostatin on adipose tissue and liver metabolism. We have looked at this with the perfused liver and perfused rat hind limb preparation and in eviscerated animals; we found no effect.

So from all the evidence that we have to date, whatever changes we see in glucose turnover appear to be due to its inhibiting the action, or secretion, of other hormones. I know of no studies looking at glucose homeostasis of isolated nervous tissue. Somatostatin will diminish the electrical potentials and electrical discharges of isolated neurons.

Dr. Wall

Somatostatin is found throughout the body. Have different structures of that hormone been found in different parts of the body?

Secondly, are there any theories as to the original use for somatostatin in the body?

Dr. Gerich

In answer to your first question about multiple forms of somatostatin: in studies of the synthesis of somatostatin by fragments of the hypothalamus and isolated islets, a larger molecular species of somatostatin has been found analogous to proinsulin and, with time, there is a transfer of tritium counts from the large molecule into a smaller molecule which has the same molecular weight and immunoreactivity as synthetic somatostatin. So there appears to be a precursor molecule.

It is possible, also, that within different areas of the body there may be different somatostatins. There is some evidence of this based on the biologic activity and immunoreactivity in following the purification of somatostatin. In some of the original studies there was a disassociation betewen immunoreactivity and biologic activity suggesting that there were perhaps multiple forms of somatostatin. But there is no hard data on this now.

Dr. Burns

I have a question. I think one of the most exciting things about the somatostatin story when it began to emerge with Dr. Guillemin in your group was the hope that it held out for better control of the erratic labile diabetic. That is, if you had a long-acting somatostatin that you could inject once a day, could you then permanently, or temporarily at least, suppress glucagon, administer insulin as before, and avoid the high peaks of hyperglycemia? Is that still a viable notion?

Dr. Gerich

Very much viable. Now, there are three groups that have confirmed a beneficial effect of somatostatin in diabetic control: my own studies, those from Dr. Pfeiffer's group in Germany, and Dr. Lundbaek's group in Denmark. A very objective means of evaluating this is the Biostator, a computerized artificial pancreas with which you can dial a blood glucose level and it will infuse sufficient insulin or glucose based on an algorithm to give you that blood glucose level. Studies by Dr. Pfeiffer's group, using this machine, indicate that when infusing somatostatin one can get better control with up to 70% reduction in insulin administered by the machine, despite the fact that the machine has to give more glucose.

Dr. Lundbaek's group has studied insulin requiring juvenile-type diabetics and adult-onset diabetics and found that in the dibetics receiving exogenous insulin diabetic control is improved, whereas in the adult onset diabetics control is worsened.

Now, this is completely expected because you have patients with marginal insulin release in whom somatostatin causes a further reduction in that insulin release which is not compensated for by the reduction in growth hormone and glucagon secretion. Regardless of what mechanism is involved, whether it be in the gut, blockade of growth hormone secretion, or glucagon secretion, studies to date indicate beneficial effects in insulin-requiring patients.

What we need now are longer-acting somatostatin analogues and perhaps more specific analogues. We would not like to induce pernicious anemia with somatostatin. We would not want to produce hypothyroidism with somatostatin. So more specific analogues will not only tell us, perhaps, how somatostatin is really working, but enable us to start some longer clinical studies. The longest ones to date have only been three days.

Dr. Klachko

Perhaps an alternative to the use of long-acting somatostatin would be achieved with an infusion mechanism. Regular somatostatin could be infused at a very slow rate from a depot reservoir and not exposed to proteolytic enzymes or peptidases, or whatever does break it down.

For this, one of the important factors would be the stability of the somatostatin molecule over long periods of time at body temperature. Has anyone looked at this?

Dr. Gerich

I can tell you if you put it in a plastic syringe and keep it at room temperature for three days without albumin or any other substance to coat the syringe, it maintains full biologic activity. At something like 10°, it will maintain its biologic activity for up to two or three weeks. Some investigators have looked at the release of somatostatin from the Alza ® mini-pump. Unfortunately, when they were looking at it they found that it was adsorbed to the inside of the pump and was not released. But this was very early in the development of the Alza pump and, perhaps, with the newer models it may be able to be released adequately.

If so, we might use one of these pumps for a prolonged period of time in an animal model for diabetes. Each pump lasts seven days. So, if one used one for six days and then implanted another one, one could have an idea of what to expect if one performed long-term administration in humans.

Dr. Brownlee

I wonder if you could clarify one point, and that is a contrast between the effects achieved by Dr. Pfeiffer, for instance, using somatostatin and the effects that one could achieve with increasing the insulin dose. Certainly, if they are equivalent, there would be no advantage to developing somatostatin analogues simply to reduce the degree of hyperglycemia, since one could do that with insulin. It is my impression that actually one is affecting the amplitude of glycemic excursion or some parameter, rather than just duplicating what you could do with more insulin.

Dr. Gerich

Yes. This is an extremely important question because if we can improve diabetic control with more insulin, or insulin used more wisely, to the same degree as with somatostatin and a lesser amount of insulin, there would be no point in developing analogues of somatostatin. But in point-of-fact, using conventional insulin, it is extremely difficult to get normalization of blood glucose values.

We performed a study that has appeared in *Diabetologia* designed to look at this. We admitted patients to our metabolic ward and tried to get them under the best possible diabetic control that we could using mixtures of regular and NPH insulin twice a day. When we had them to the point where we were causing hypoglycemia, we diminished the insulin and studied them for two days; then we diminished the insulin further while infusing somatostatin. We found that using less insulin we got better control than with what we thought was our optimal insulin levels.

Dr. Burns

Yesterday I asked Dr. Levine what he thought about the formulation that Unger had published in the New England Journal recently and he deferred the question until today's presentation. I wonder if I could ask that again, Dr. Levine. Specifically, what do you think of this formulation wherein these three hormones--insulin, glucagon, and somatostatin--are said to be orchestrating the flow of nutrient fuel into the circulation and out of the circulation?

Dr. Levine

I can only answer that I am not ready to formulate that--not with all the organs in which somatostatin is found. I think we should wait.

Dr. Burns

He's a hard man to pin down.

INSULIN RESISTANT SYNDROMES IN HUMANS

Robert S. Bar, Michele Muggeo, and Jesse Roth[1]

Division of Endocrinology and Metabolism
University of Iowa; Iowa City, IA 52242
Diabetes Branch; NIAMDD; NIH; Bethesda, MD 20014

INTRODUCTION

Clinical states of insulin resistance are characterized by elevated circulating levels of insulin and resistance to the action of exogenous insulin (Berson and Yalow, 1970). In some states of insulin resistance, delivery of insulin to target tissues is impaired; however, in most, the delivery of insulin to its peripheral target tissues is normal and the resistance results from peripheral antagonism to the action of insulin. Several recent studies have examined the interaction of insulin with its target cell receptors in clinical conditions of diminished sensitivity to insulin (Bar and Roth, 1977; Kahn, Megyesi, Bar, Eastman, and Flier, 1977). These studies have demonstrated that both the concentration and the affinity of the insulin receptors undergo wide fluctuation under numerous biologically relevant conditions. Several conditions were characterized by decreases in the concentration of receptors, with the decrease in receptor concentration related to the severity of the insulin resistance. In other conditions, changes in receptor affinity were predominant and were unrelated to the environmental insulin concentration. Taken together, these studies indicate that the insulin receptor is a major site for the regulation of target cell responsiveness *in vivo*.

MECHANISM OF INSULIN RESISTANCE IN MAN

Mechanism of Insulin Action

Before discussing insulin resistance, it is helpful to review

[1]Supported, in part, by a grant from the Iowa Affiliate of the American Diabetes Association.

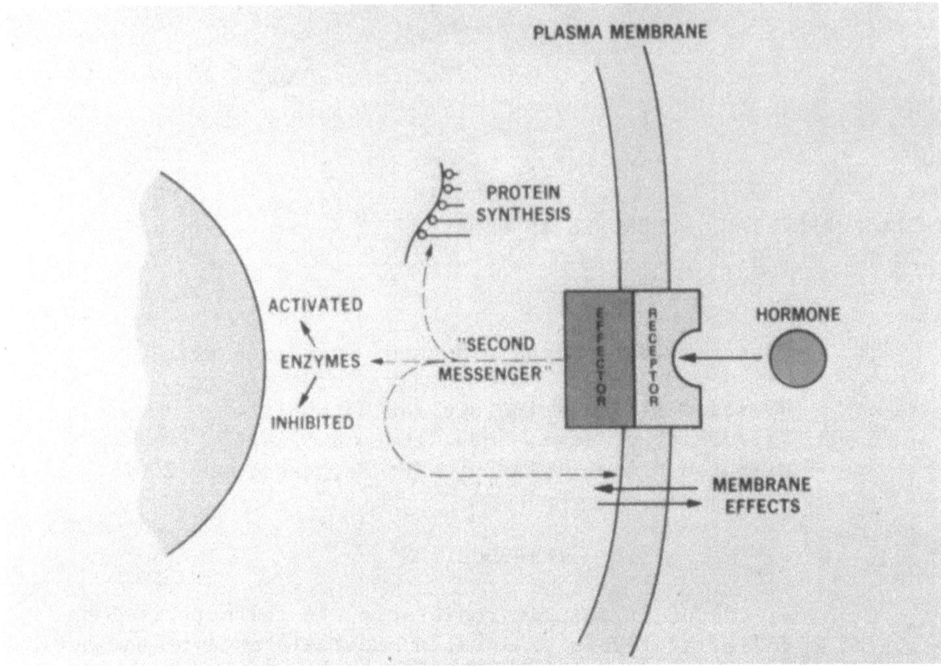

Figure 1. Schematic representation of insulin action.

first the mechanisms of insulin action (Figure 1). After release from the pancreatic *beta* cell, insulin enters the vascular compartment where it circulates in a free or unbound state. Once at the target tissue, insulin initiates its action by first binding to specific sites on the outer plasma membrane, known as receptors (Desbuquois and Cuatrecasas, 1973). The hormone-receptor complexes then initiate a series of intracellular processes which result in the characteristic effects of insulin. With this scheme of insulin action in mind, it is apparent that there are several potential defects that could result in a state of insulin resistance. These defects could occur before insulin reaches its target tissue or, alternatively, could result from abnormalities at the level of the target tissue itself (Table 1). As alluded to in the introduction, most states of insulin resistance result from defects at the target tissue itself indicating the presence of either receptor or postreceptor defects. Unfortunately, we cannot accurately measure the several intracellular processes required for insulin action. However, in the last several years methodology has been developed to assess the interaction of insulin with its specific receptors on target tissues. Such methodology has been successfully employed to evaluate insulin-receptor interaction in several clinical condi-

Table 1. POTENTIAL MECHANISMS OF INSULIN RESISTANCE

I. Defects proximal to the Target Cell
   1. insulin biologically inactive
   2. insulin bound to serum proteins (*e.g.*, insulin antibodies)
   3. increased degradation rate of insulin
   4. increased proportion of proinsulin

II. Defects at the Target Cell
   1. receptor
      - decreased concentration
      - decreased affinity
   2. postreceptor
      - abnormalities of transmembrane and intracellular processes

tions of altered sensitivity to insulin.

The remainder of this discussion will focus on two clinical states of insulin resistance in which alterations at the level of the insulin receptor appear to play a major role in the pathogenesis of the observed insulin-resistant states. The two conditions are obesity and the syndromes of insulin resistance and acanthosis nigricans.

OBESITY

Obesity is the most common and, perhaps, best studied form of hormone resistance in man (Rabinowitz, 1970). As an example, we will first present laboratory data for one such insulin-resistant patient (Figure 2). During glucose tolerance testing, plasma glucose levels were essentially normal (Figure 2a). After several weeks of low-calorie diet, there was a slight decrease in plasma glucose levels, but they were still within the normal range. In contrast, the insulin responses during the glucose tolerance test

Figure 2. Glucose tolerance tests and intravenous insulin tolerance tests in an obese patient in the basal (fed) state and after several weeks of low-calorie diet. Plasma glucose responses (2a) and plasma insulin responses (2b) to 100 g ingestion of glucose are plotted. Shaded areas represent the ranges of normal. Plasma glucose responses to intravenous insulin (0.1 U/kg body weight) are given for an obese patient and normal (2c).

← *Figure 2a*

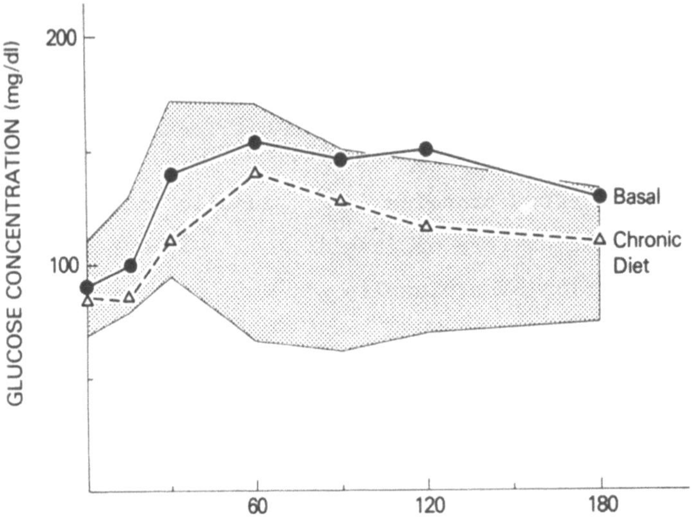

Figure 2b →

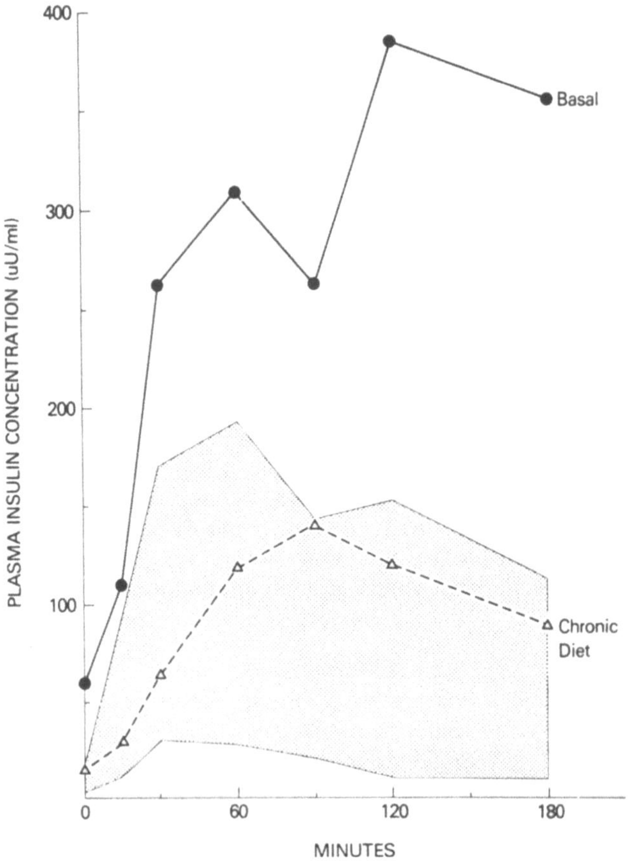

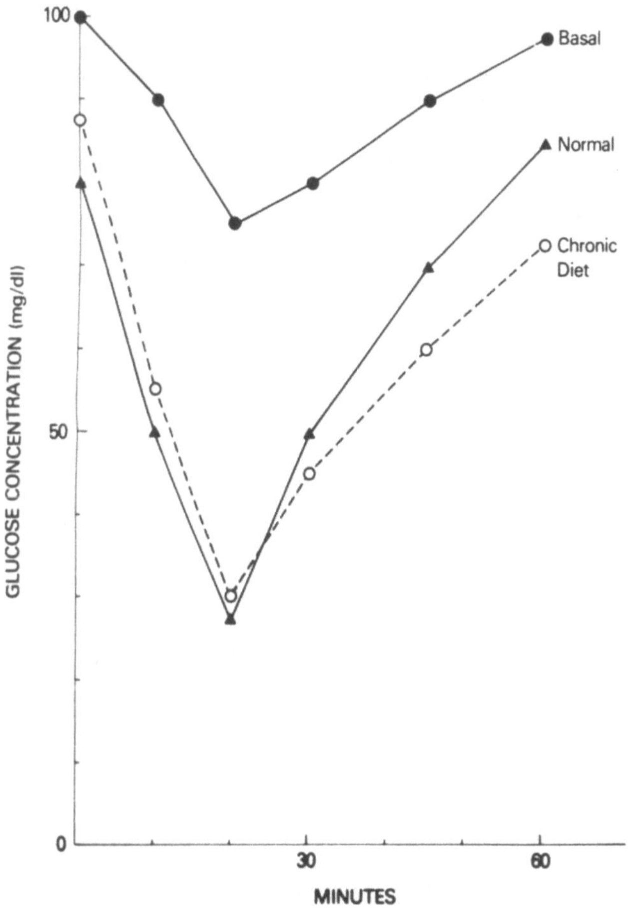

← Figure 2c

were markedly abnormal (Figure 2b). In the basal (fed) state, circulating insulin levels were three to five times greater than normal. After several weeks of low-calorie diet, endogenous insulin levels fell to the normal range. This patient also demonstrated impaired responsiveness to exogenously administered insulin (Figure 2c). After several weeks of chronic dieting, response to administered insulin was now normal, illustrating the reversible nature of the insulin resistance in obesity.

Insulin resistance, such as seen in this obese patient, can be caused by defects proximal to the target cell or at the level of the target cell (Table 1). In obesity, defects proximal to the target cell do not account for the insulin resistance. Specifically, the circulating insulin is biologically active and is not bound to serum proteins such as insulin antibodies. There is neither an increased rate of insulin degradation nor an increased proportion of proinsulin, which reacts well in the radioimmunoassay for insulin but has little biological activity. These findings suggest that in obesity, defects at the target cell must occur and, in fact, several studies have directly documented end-organ resistance in obesity (Rabinowitz and Zierler, 1961).

INSULIN RECEPTORS IN OBESITY

Two types of human tissue, circulating monocytes and adipose tissue, have served as sources of insulin receptors for study of human obesity. The fat cell and monocyte have several identical physicochemical properties relative to insulin binding. These properties include (1) a pH dependence of binding, (2) temperature dependence of binding, (3) curvilinear Scatchard plots, and (4) the kinetic equivalent of negative cooperativity, *i.e.*, acceleration of the dissociation rate of receptor-bound insulin by unlabeled insulin. Most importantly, both monocytes and fat cells show similar inhibition of ^{125}I-insulin binding by insulins of differing biopotencies. These several physicochemical properties are also shared by the insulin receptors of liver and muscle, the two tissues most relevant to overall glucose homeostasis *in vivo*.

In human obesity, results from both receptor sources are essentially similar; therefore, all subsequent data of insulin binding refer to monocyte studies (Bar, Gorden, Roth, Kahn, and De Meyts, 1976; Harrison, Martin, and Melick, 1976). The insulin binding to human monocytes from several obese patients is illustrated in Figure 3. Some obese patients have normal insulin binding, whereas others show variable degrees of impairment of insulin binding. When these data were quantitatively analyzed by Scatchard plots (Scatchard, 1949) and average affinity profiles (De Meyts and Roth, 1975), it became apparent that the decreases in insulin binding were due solely to a decrease in the concentration of insulin receptors. By several criteria, these receptors had normal affinity, but were only reduced in number. Furthermore, when the binding data were compared to the clinical state of the patient, it was found that those obese patients with the lowest insulin binding and the lowest receptor concentrations had the greatest insulin resistance. Obese patients without clinical evidence of insulin resistance had normal insulin binding and normal concentrations of insulin receptors on their cells. This relationship between receptor concentration and insulin resistance (as determined by circulating insulin levels) is further illustrated for a group of obese patients in Figure 4. Again, patients with more pronounced insulin resistance, such as patient E, have the lowest receptor concentration; patients with lesser degrees of insulin resistance, such as patient A, have normal concentrations of receptors.

We have previously indicated that the insulin resistance is reversed by chronic dieting. Chronic diet also induces commensu-

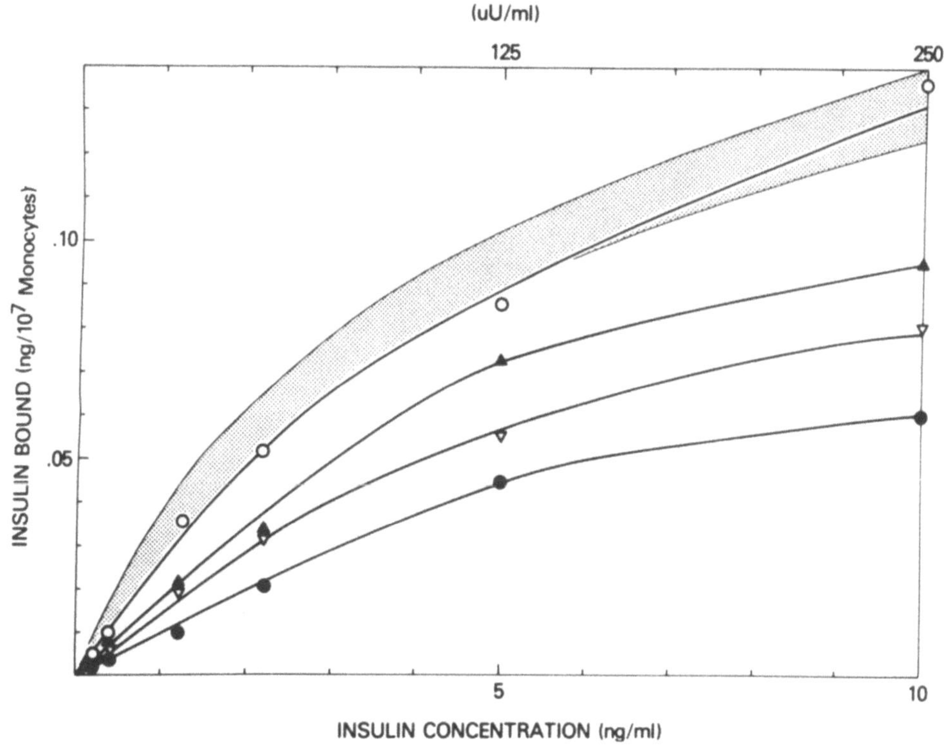

Figure 3. Insulin binding to circulating monocytes from four obese patients. Bound insulin (ng/10^7 cells) is plotted as a function of total insulin concentration in the incubation assay. Shaded area is the range of normal. Data in this figure and in Figures 4, 5, 6, and 7 have been adapted from Bar et al. (1976) with permission.

rate changes in insulin binding (Figure 5). In the basal or fed state this obese patient had decreased binding of insulin to his circulating monocytes. After ten weeks of a 600-calorie diet he lost approximately 10 *kg* in weight, lowered his plasma insulin levels and, as seen in Figure 5, increased insulin binding into the normal range. When such binding data were quantitatively analyzed, it was found that the increase in insulin binding was due to an increase in the concentration of insulin receptors. The effects of chronic diet on plasma insulin and insulin receptor concentration are illustrated for several obese patients in Figure 6. In the basal state, all patients had significant insulin resistance, as documented by intravenous insulin tolerance tests and endogenous hyperinsulinemia and decreased concentrations of insulin receptors on their monocytes. After several weeks to several months of chronic dieting, they all lowered their plasma insulin levels and increased receptor concentrations towards normal. Thus, the re-

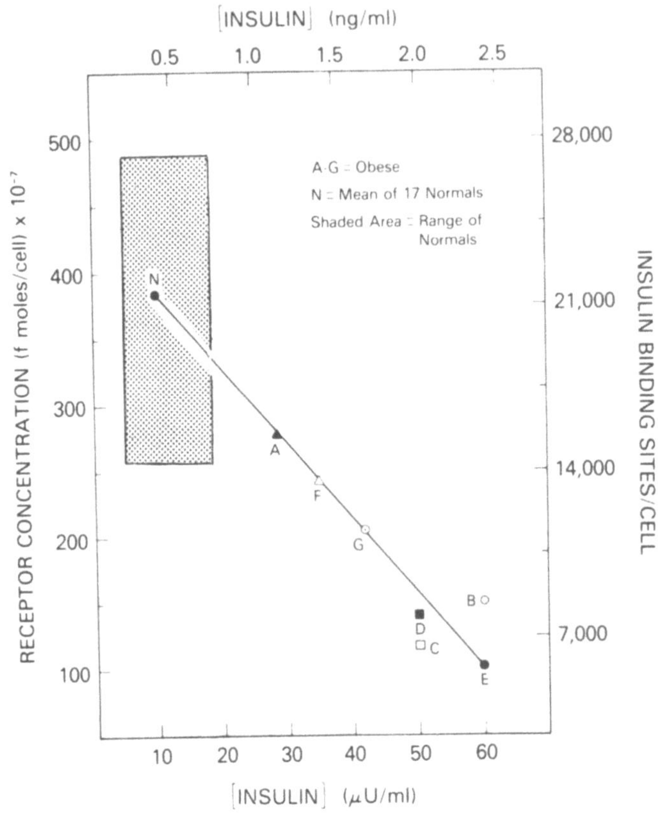

Figure 4. Correlation of plasma insulin concentration and receptor concentration in monocytes from obese patients. The shaded rectangle represents the range of normal.

versal of clinical insulin resistance with chronic diet was associated with an increase in the concentration of insulin receptors.

The data presented in Figures 4 and 6 indicate an inverse relationship between insulin receptor concentration and plasma levels of insulin. This relationship was also observed in rodent models of obesity (Soll, Kahn, Neville, and Roth 1975). These rodent models include genetic forms of obesity (ob/ob and db/db mice) as well as acquired obesity (mice treated with gold thioglucose). As in human obesity, these mice are hyperinsulinemic and resistant to the effects of exogenously administered insulin. Additionally, they have been shown to have a decreased concentration of insulin receptors on all tissues studied thus far, including insulin receptors from muscle, liver, fat, and thymic lymphocytes. The magnitude of the decrease in receptor concentration was directly proportional to the level of plasma insulin (Figure 7, center).

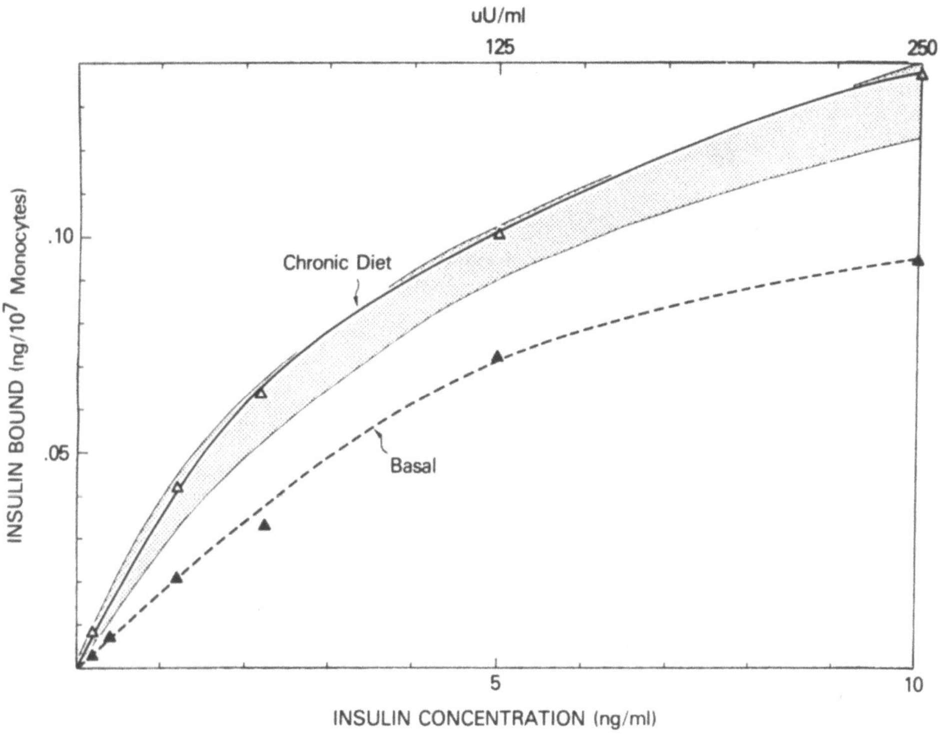

Figure 5. The effect of long-term, low-calorie diet on insulin binding to monocytes from an insulin-resistant, obese patient. The shaded area is the normal range.

When such mice were acutely fasted for 24 hours, plasma insulin levels fell and insulin binding and insulin receptor concentration increased towards normal. When the same mice were fasted for 24 hours, but supplemented with exogenous insulin to maintain their hyperinsulinemia, insulin binding did not increase, suggesting that insulin, *per se*, may have a direct regulatory role on its own receptor.

The effect of insulin on its receptor has been most clearly demonstrated in cultured cell systems (Gavin, Roth, Neville, De Meyts, and Buell, 1974). When human lymphoblastoid cells of the IM-9 line were grown in the presence of insulin, the concentration of insulin receptors was reduced, with the receptor decrease proportional to the concentration of ambient insulin (Figure 7). Such *in vitro* studies demonstrate directly that insulin can modulate its own receptor.

The clinical and laboratory data that we have thus far presented are most consistent with the pathogenesis of obesity out-

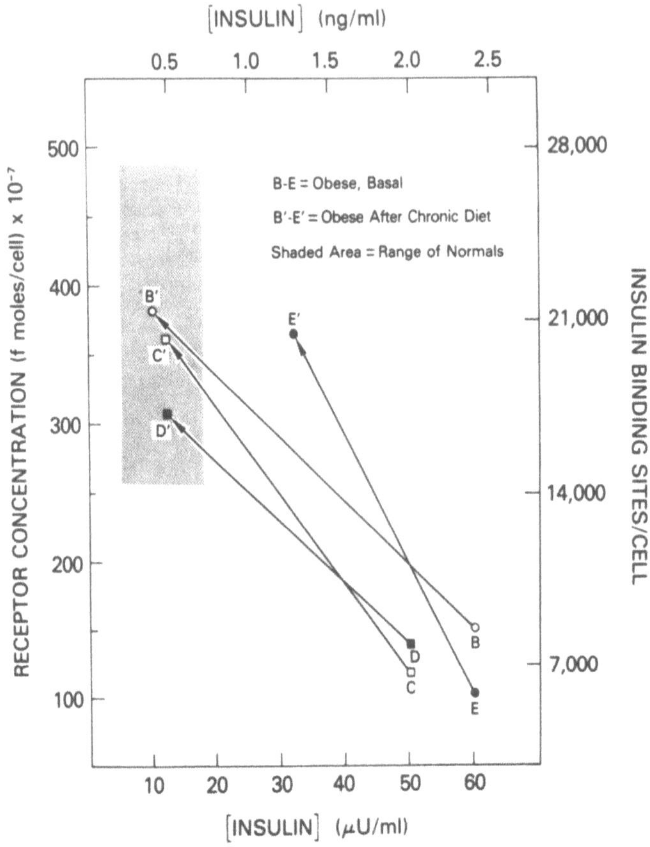

Figure 6. Relationship between insulin receptor concentration on monocytes and plasma insulin levels for four obese patients before and after chronic low-calorie diet.

lined in Figure 8. In this formulation, overeating is the primary etiologic agent. The increased food intake causes increased blood glucose and plasma insulin levels. The chronic hyperinsulinemia results in a "down regulation" of insulin receptors and a state of insulin resistance. When food intake is curtailed, plasma insulin levels fall, receptor concentration normalizes, and insulin resistance abates.

THE SYNDROMES OF ACANTHOSIS NIGRICANS AND INSULIN RESISTANCE

In 1961, Field, Johnson, and Herring described a young female with acanthosis nigricans and severe insulin resistance (Field, Johnson, and Herring, 1961). We have had the opportunity to study 11 patients with marked similarities to this patient (Flier, Kahn,

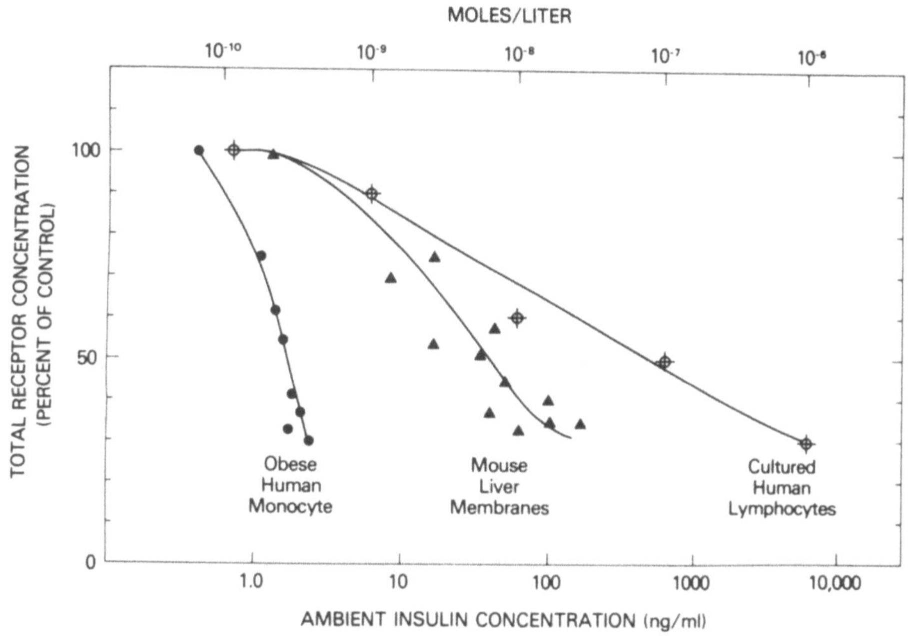

Figure 7. Insulin receptor concentrations as a function of ambient insulin concentration in the obese humans, obese mice, and cultured human lymphocytes. For humans, 100% receptor concentration represents the mean value obtained in thin controls and for the mice 100% value is the mean receptor concentration of thin mice.

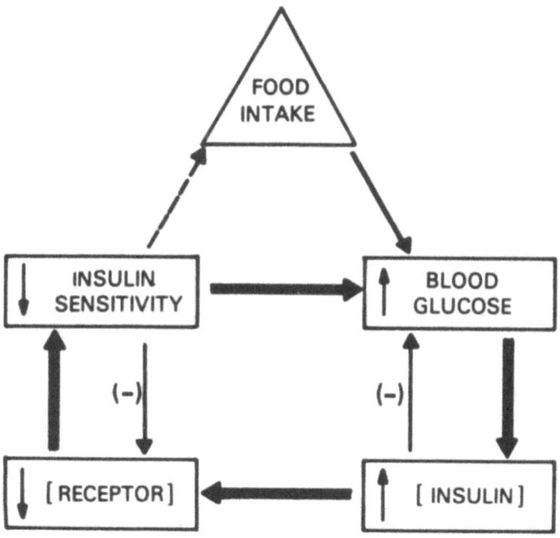

Figure 8. Pathogenesis of insulin resistance in obesity.

Roth, and Bar, 1975; Kahn, Flier, Bar, Archer, Gorden, Martin, and Roth, 1976). Common features among these 11 patients are outlined in Table 2. All are markedly resistant to the action of both endogenous and exogenous insulin. In general, their insulin resistance is several-fold greater than that found in human obesity. Likewise, insulin binding to their monocytes tends to be much lower than previously noted in the obese patients (Figure 9). For an individual patient, the greater the clinical resistance to insulin the more pronounced the insulin binding defect.

When the clinical and laboratory features of these patients were analyzed, they segregated into two distinct groups, designated Type A and Type B patients. The Type A patients were younger females characterized by signs and symptoms of excess androgen. The four Type A patients whom we have studied ranged in age from 12 to 18 years. All were hirsute and had polycystic ovarian disease. The Type B patients were older with signs and symptoms of autoimmune disease including positive antinuclear antibodies, anti-DNA antibodies, increased erythrocyte sedimentation rate, increased concentrations of *gamma* globulins, decreased white blood cell counts, alopecia, and proteinuria. All seven Type B patients have been shown by Dr. Jeffrey Flier to have circulating antibodies that block the binding of insulin to its own receptors (anti-receptor antibodies). In an individual patient, the titer of anti-receptor antibody correlates with both the degree of clinical insulin resistance and the degree of impairment of insulin binding

Table 2. THE SYNDROMES OF INSULIN RESISTANCE AND ACANTHOSIS NIGRICANS

1. Acquired defect, variable age at onset
2. Female preponderance - 10 to 1
3. Acanthosis Nigricans (8/11) - variable severity
4. Extreme resistance to endogenous and exogenous insulin
5. Hyperinsulinemia - 10 to 100 times normal
6. Absence of known causes of insulin resistance
   - no, or low, titer of anti-insulin antibodies
   - no obesity or lipoatrophy
   - no Cushing's or acromegaly
7. Variable glucose tolerance
8. Markedly reduced insulin binding to its specific receptor
   - 1 to 50% of normal

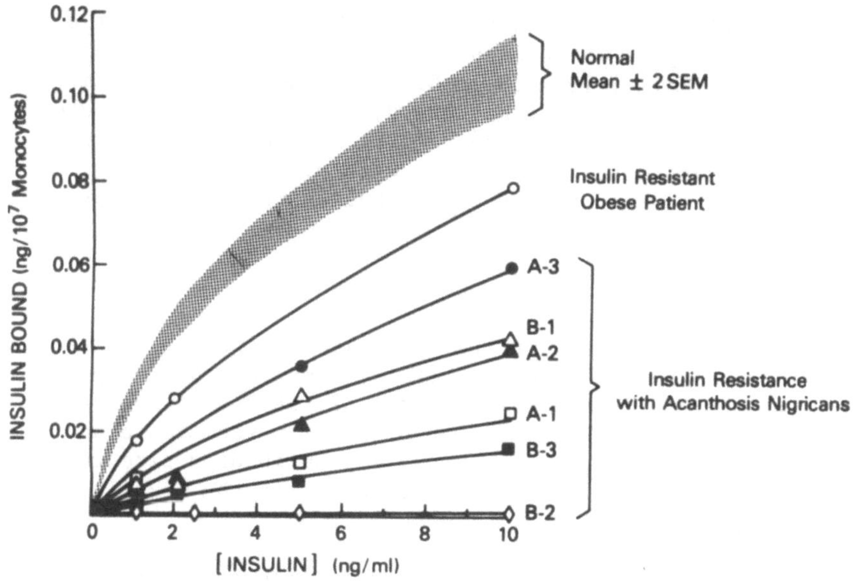

Figure 9. Insulin binding to monocytes of patients with insulin resistance and acanthosis nigricans. A study of an insulin-resistant, obese patient is shown for comparison. The shaded area is the range of normals (adapted from Kahn et al., 1976).

to that patient's monocytes. In addition to blocking the binding of insulin to its receptors, some anti-receptor antibodies have intrinsic insulin-like activity. The characteristics of these anti-receptor antibodies are summarized in Table 3.

Circulating auto-antibodies that block hormone binding to its receptor are not unique to the syndromes that we have just described. In fact, two common entities, Graves' disease and

Table 3. CHARACTERISTICS OF BINDING INHIBITOR

1. Inhibits insulin binding on wide variety of tissues
   - hepatocytes, adipocytes, cultured lymphocytes and mammary cells, avian erythrocytes
2. Has no effect on binding of other hormones
3. Immunoglobulin by several criteria
   - ammonium sulfate precipitation
   - gel filtration
   - DEAE chromatography
   - specific immunoprecipitation

myasthenia gravis, are also characterized by the presence of circulating anti-receptor antibodies (Bender, Rengel, Engle, Daniels, and Vogel, 1975; Smith, 1974). In Graves' disease, both stimulatory and blocking antibodies that are directed against the receptor for thyroid-stimulating hormone (TSH) have been demonstrated in the sera of patients. In patients with myasthenia gravis, antibodies directed against the acetylcholine receptor are present.

SUMMARY AND CONCLUSIONS

We have presented data on the mechanism of insulin resistance in two clinical states. In one, obesity, insulin itself appears to play a major role in the pathogenesis of the resistance state. In a second condition, the syndromes of insulin resistance and acanthosis nigricans (Type B), circulating antibodies directed against the insulin receptor appear to result in the insulin-resistant state.

We should emphasize that the status of insulin receptors has been carefully investigated in other states of altered insulin sensitivity. In several conditions there are marked changes in both the affinity and the concentration of insulin receptors which are unrelated to either the ambient insulin level or the presence of receptor antibodies, indicating that there are several as yet unknown mediators of the insulin-receptor interaction. Secondly, in several states of marked insulin resistance, insulin receptors have been found to be normal, suggesting the presence of postreceptor or intracellular defects in the target cells which cause the insulin resistance. In the near future, we look forward to the elucidation of these other mediators of the insulin-receptor interaction as well as to the development of methodology that will enable detailed assessment of intracellular processes necessary for insulin action.

REFERENCES

Bar, R.S., Gorden, P., Roth J., Kahn, C.R., and De Meyts, P. 1976. Fluctuations in the affinity and concentration of insulin receptors on circulating monocytes of obese patients. *J. Clin. Invest.* **58**:1123-1135.

Bar, R.S. and Roth, J. 1977. Insulin receptor status in disease states of man. *Arch. Int. Med.* **137**:474-481.

Bender, A.N., Rengel, S.P., Engle, W.K., Daniels, M.P., and Vogel, Z. 1975. Myasthenia gravis: A serum factor blocking acetylcholine receptors of the human neuromuscular function. *Lancet* **1**:607-609.

Berson, S.A. and Yalow, R.S. 1970. Insulin "antagonists" and insulin resistance. p. 389. IN M. Ellenberg and H. Rifkin

(Eds.) *Diabetes mellitus: Theory and practice.* New York: McGraw-Hill.

De Meyts, P. and Roth, J. 1975. Cooperativity in ligand binding. A new graphic analysis. *Biochem. Biophys. Res. Commun.* **66**: 1118-1126.

Desbuquois, B. and Cuatrecasas, P. 1973. Insulin receptors. *Ann. Rev. Med.* **24**:233-240.

Field, J.B., Johnson, P., and Herring, B. 1961. Insulin-resistant diabetes associated with increased endogenous plasma insulin followed by complete remission. *J. Clin. Invest.* **40**: 1672-1683.

Flier, J.S., Kahn, C.R., Roth, J., and Bar, R.S. 1975. Antibodies that impair insulin receptor binding in an unusual diabetic syndrome with severe insulin resistance. *Science* **190**:63-65.

Gavin, J.R. III, Roth, J., Neville, D.M., Jr., De Meyts, P., and Buell, D.M. 1974. Insulin-dependent regulation of insulin receptor concentrations. A direct demonstration in cell culture. *Proc. Natl. Acad. Sci.* USA **71**:84-88.

Harrison, L.C., Martin, F.I.R., and Melick, R.A. 1976. Correlation between insulin receptor binding in isolated fat cells and insulin sensitivity in obese human subjects. *J. Clin. Invest.* **58**:1435-1441.

Kahn, C.R., Flier, J.S., Bar, R.S., Archer, J.A., Gorden, P., Martin, M., and Roth, J. 1976. The syndromes of insulin resistance and acanthosis nigricans. *N. Eng. J. Med.* **294**: 739-745.

Kahn, C.R., Megyesi, K., Bar, R.S., Eastman, R.C., and Flier, J.S. 1977. Receptors for peptide hormones. *Ann. Int. Med.* **86**:205-219.

Rabinowitz, D. 1970. Some endocrine and metabolic aspects of obesity. *Ann. Rev. Med.* **21**:241-258.

Rabinowitz, D. and Zierler, K.L. 1961. Forearm metabolism in obesity and its response to intra-arterial insulin. *Lancet* **2**:690-692.

Scatchard, G. 1949. The attractions of proteins for small molecules and ions. *Ann. NY Acad. Sci.* **51**:660-672.

Smith, B.R. 1974. Thyroid-stimulating immunoglobulins in Graves' disease. *Lancet* **2**:427-431.

Soll, A.H., Kahn, C.R., Neville, D.M., Jr., and Roth, J. 1975. Insulin receptor deficiency in genetic and acquired obesity. *J. Clin. Invest.* **56**:769-780.

DISCUSSION FOLLOWING DR. BAR'S TALK

Dr. Steffes

You demonstrated very high levels of insulin in people with extreme insulin resistance. How long do these people continue producing excess amounts of insulin? Everyone talks teleologically about islet exhaustion in juvenile diabetes. Does this syndrome give us information with regard to that hypothesis?

Dr. Bar

In a five- to six-year follow-up we have not observed pancreatic exhaustion in either the Type A or Type B, but this may only reflect the short period of observation. The Type A patients tend to remain relatively stable in terms of their insulin resistance and their own insulin levels. On the other hand, the Type B patients have shown marked changes in their insulin resistance, insulin binding defect on their circulating cells and in the character of their circulating anti-receptor antibodies. Three Type B patients have actually developed hypoglycemia associated with improvement in insulin binding to their circulating monocytes (Bar, Flier, and Jarrett, 1977; Flier, Bar, Muggeo, Kahn, Roth, and Gorden, 1978). At present, we are not sure of the mechanisms of these changes. In any case, it is probably best to view any findings in the Type A and Type B patients in their own context and not extrapolate to the more common forms of diabetes.

Dr. Jackson

For the past 20 years we have been performing serial standardized oral glucose tolerance tests (O.G.T.T.'s) on the siblings of our children with overt diabetes. We also have established norms for blood sugar and serum insulin levels during O.G.T.T.'s in normal pre- and postpubescent boys and girls. About 15% of the siblings of the children with overt diabetes have been found to have abnormal O.G.T.T.'s. We were surprised to find definite hyperinsulinemia with normoglycemia in a number of nonobese siblings, but few, if any, of these research subjects have progressed to overt insulin-dependent diabetes during adolescence. We also have observed that with cessation of linear growth, the O.G.T.T.'s tend to improve rather than become more abnormal. We have found that siblings with abnormal insulin as well as abnormal blood sugar curves are more likely to progress to overt diabetes during their prepubescent growth spurts.

Dr. Bar

Thank you.

Dr. Gerich

This is related to Dr. Steffes' question. I noticed in one of the slides containing the results of the oral glucose tolerance tests and insulin levels in the patients with acanthosis nigricans that the people with the highest insulin levels had the most normal glucose tolerance test. It would seem that the major determinant of whether the insulin resistance leads to diabetes is not the insulin resistance *per se*, but the ability of the *beta* cell to compensate for it.

Dr. Bar

Your assessment of that slide is perfectly correct. Those patients that had the highest insulin levels tended to have most normal blood glucose levels. I would agree that the major determinant of hyperglycemia appears to be the ability of the *beta* cell to produce insulin and, therefore, compensate for the peripheral insulin resistance. We do not know the cause of the insulin resistance in the Type A patients. However, if we use graded insulin tolerance tests as an index of insulin resistance, then the most accurate reflector of insulin resistance is <u>not</u> the blood glucose nor the circulating level of insulin, but the magnitude of the monocyte-binding defect in the Type A patients, whereas, in the Type B patients, both the monocyte-binding defect and the titer of anti-receptor antibody accurately reflect the level of insulin resistance.

Dr. Levine

Dr. Bar, have you or anybody in your group tested the metabolic effects of adding receptor antibodies to cell systems? For example, the adipose tissue, if you added the receptor antibody and, therefore, effectively removed the receptor, could you duplicate what Kuhne found for trypsin? In other words, does the glucose influx increase without added insulin?

Dr. Bar

Dr. Ronald Kahn at the NIH has extensively tested sera and immunoglobulin fractions from sera of Type B patients for their ability to stimulate glucose oxidation in isolated adipocytes as well as ability to block insulin binding in the same cell type (Kahn, Baird, Flier, and Jarrett, 1977). He found that certain sera primarily blocked binding of insulin to its receptor <u>without</u> stimulating glucose oxidation, other sera were more potent <u>in</u>

their ability to stimulate glucose oxidation and, finally, some sera were equipotent in their ability to stimulate glucose oxidation and inhibit insulin binding. These data, coupled with other findings of Jeff Flier, Len Harrison, and David Jarrett suggest the presence of a heterogenous group of anti-receptor antibodies which recognize different regions of the insulin receptor. The separation of the specific anti-receptor antibodies is presently being attempted, since such antibodies have obvious importance as research probes in studying the nature of the insulin receptor.

Dr. Werner

In any cellular control mechanism the rate-limiting step is usually the slowest step, the so-called bottleneck. We have been told, over and over, how much excess receptors we have on the cells where 5% to 10% perhaps are needed for the maximal effect. With such an excess of receptors, how could this be the rate-limiting step?

Dr. Bar

In the case of spare receptors, a decrease in the concentration of insulin receptors would result in a rightward shift of the dose-response curve for insulin, providing that all steps distal to the hormone-receptor interaction remain unchanged. As an example, let's take some actual data for glucose oxidation in rat adipocytes (Kono and Barham, 1971). In these cells, maximal levels of glucose oxidation occur when only 10% of the total cell receptors are occupied by insulin. When the concentration of insulin receptors are reduced by exposure to trypsin, the dose-response curve for insulin-stimulated oxidation shifts to the right, *i.e.*, maximal effects of insulin do occur but require higher concentrations of insulin, which in turn are needed to form the necessary number of hormone receptor complexes.

The physiological relevance of receptor loss, such as seen in obesity, is not known for certain. If all other pre- and postreceptor steps remain intact, we would expect the insulin-mediated processes that exhibit "spare receptors" to behave similarly to the isolated adipocytes just mentioned. Again, in such a circumstance a maximal effect of insulin could conceivably occur but would require higher than normal concentrations of circulating insulin (Bar, Harrison, Muggeo, Gorden, Kahn, and Roth, 1978; Kono and Barham, 1971).

DISCUSSION REFERENCES

Bar, R.S., Flier, J.S., and Jarrett, D.B. 1977. Hypoglycemia and proliferation of low affinity insulin receptors in a patient with anti-receptor antibodies. *Diabetes* **26**:354. (Abstr.)

Bar, R.S., Harrison, L.C., Muggeo, M.M., Gordon, P., Kahn, C.R., and Roth, J. 1979. Regulation of insulin receptors in normal and abnormal physiology in humans. *Adv. Intern. Med.* (in press).

Flier, J.S., Bar, R.S., Muggeo, M.M., Kahn, C.R., Roth, J., and Gorden, P. 1978. The evolving course of patients with insulin receptor autoantibodies: Spontaneous remission or receptor proliferation with hypoglycemia. *J. Clin. Endocrin. Metab.* **47**:985-995.

Kahn, C.R., Baird, K., Flier, J.S., and Jarrett, D.B. 1977. Effects of autoantibodies to the insulin receptor on isolated adipocytes. Studies of insulin binding and insulin action. *J. Clin. Invest.* **60**:1094-1106.

Kono, T. and Barham, F.W. 1971. The relationship between the insulin binding capacity of fat cells and the cellular response to insulin. Studies with intact and trypsin-treated fat cells. *J. Biol. Chem.* **246**:6210-6216.

BIOCHEMICAL DERANGEMENTS IN DIABETES MELLITUS

R.S. Clements, Jr.[1]

Diabetes Research and Training Center
University of Alabama School of Medicine
Birmingham, AL 35294

OUTLINE

I. Introduction

II. Abnormal protein glycosylation

- A. Glomerular basement membrane
- B. Serum glycoproteins
- C. Platelet proteins
- D. Hemoglobin

III. Polyol pathway

- A. Lens
- B. Nerve
- C. Aorta

IV. Abnormal myoinositol metabolism

- A. Myoinositol metabolism in the human with diabetes mellitus
- B. Nerve myoinositol metabolism

V. Summary and conclusions

INTRODUCTION

During the fifty-sixth year since the discovery of insulin, most physicians who are concerned with the care of the diabetic

[1]Original research supported by grants from the Juvenile Diabetes Foundation, Veterans Administration, and grants RR-32 and AM-21065 from the National Institutes of Health.

have become more willing to accept the possibility that the development of diabetic complications may be related to the metabolic consequences of hyperglycemia. Since those tissues which require insulin for the intracellular transport of glucose (*i.e.*, muscle and fat) appear to be relatively immune to the ravages of diabetes, current research into the mechanisms by which an elevated glucose concentration could result in cellular damage has focused upon the so-called "noninsulin-dependent pathways of glucose metabolism." Obviously, this term implies that, whereas these pathways are not directly activated by insulin, the hyperglycemia which results from insulin deficiency does foster their activation. It is the purpose of this review to consider certain of these pathways and the roles which they have been speculated to play in the development of diabetic complications.

ABNORMAL PROTEIN GLYCOSYLATION

Glomerular Basement Membrane

One of the most exciting areas of research into diabetic complications is concerned with abnormal glycosylation of proteins in the diabetic. A relationship between the abnormal addition of glucose molecules to protein and the development of diabetic glomerulosclerosis was first postulated by Dr. Robert Spiro of the Joslin Research Laboratories (Beisswenger and Spiro, 1970). He observed that basement membrane material isolated from human renal glomeruli consisted of a group of collagen-like glycoproteins. This material was found to differ from collagen, in that it contained a much greater fractional content of carbohydrate. The carbohydrate molecules attached to the peptide backbone were found to be of two varieties: a heteropolysaccharide consisting of sialic acid, fucose, galactose, mannose, and N-acetyl-glucosamine which was attached to an asparagine residue, and a smaller disaccharide subunit consisting of one glucose and one galactose molecule attached to an hydroxylysine residue. He observed that glomeruli obtained from longstanding diabetics were larger and contained an increased amount of basement membrane material. Furthermore, the basement membrane of the diabetic was abnormal, in that it contained an increased ratio of hydroxylated lysine to nonhydroxylated lysine residues and that there was an increased amount of hydroxylysine-linked disaccharide side chains.

Since Kefalides has demonstrated that the addition of carbohydrate side-chains to the precursors of basement membrane material appears to be rate-limiting in their export from the cell (Grant, Kefalides, and Prockop, 1972), Spiro speculated further that abnormally rapid rates of glycosylation could account, in part, for an increase in the rate of formation of the glomerular basement membrane of the diabetic. Finally, he speculated that the increased proportion of bulky carbohydrate side-chains could interfere with the packing of the basement membrane material leading to an abnormally thickened and porous glomerular basement membrane.

To investigate these possibilities more directly, he studied the activity of the glucosyltransferase enzyme in the kidney which is responsible for the addition of the glucose molecule to the hydroxylysine-linked galactose molecule of the basement membrane precursor. He observed that with increasing age, the activity of this enzyme progressively decreased in the nondiabetic rat. In contrast, in the alloxan-diabetic rat this enzyme activity was found to increase with age. Furthermore, when he carefully treated the diabetic rats with insulin, he was able to restore their renal glucosyltransferase activity to normal. That experimental diabetes results in increased rates of lysine incorporation and hydroxylation in the glomerular basement membrane has also been demonstrated (Cohen and Vogt, 1972; Khalifa and Cohen, 1975).

These studies suggest that the glomerular basement membrane thickening which is observed in diabetic glomerulosclerosis could be due to an increase in the enzyme activity responsible for the glycosylation of the basement membrane precursor and that this increase is the direct result of either insulin deficiency or the resultant hyperglycemia. That hyperglycemia, rather than insulin deficiency, may be the culprit was subsequently suggested by *in vitro* studies which demonstrated that, whereas insulin had no effect upon the carbohydrate metabolism of the isolated glomerulus, hyperglycemia markedly increased the rate of incorporation of radioactive glucose into the glomerular basement membrane (Wahl, Deppermann, Deschner, Fuchs, and Rexroth, 1973).

Although this biochemical scheme has obvious appeal for those of us who believe that small blood vessel disease may be a consequence of exposure of the tissues of the diabetic to elevated glucose concentrations, more recent studies have cast some doubt upon its validity. Neither Kefalides (1975) nor Westberg and Michael (1973) were able to confirm the abnormal chemical composition of the glomerular basement membrane material from human diabetics. Similarly, in the glomerulus of the rat with streptozotocin diabetes, Beisswenger was unable to detect any chemical abnormality nor could he detect an increased rate of lysine incorporation into basement membrane material or an increased rate of its subsequent hydroxylation (Beisswenger, 1976). In addition, recent studies suggest that decreased rates of glycoprotein catabolism deserve equal consideration as possible mechanisms which may be involved in the pathogenesis of diabetic microvascular disease (Fushimi and Tarui, 1976). Therefore, any firm conclusions concerning the biochemical mechanisms responsible for the development of diabetic glomerular disease must be held in abeyance for the present.

Serum Glycoproteins

Over the last decade, it has become apparent that the diabetic synthesizes an increased amount of protein-bound carbohydrate in the liver and maintains elevated levels of several serum glycoproteins--in particular, the α-globulins (McMillan, 1972). Although the mechanism responsible for the increased hepatic glycoprotein production has not been elucidated, relationships between the effects of increased serum glycoprotein concentrations and increased blood viscosity have been proposed. It is possible that such changes in blood viscosity could be related to altered circulatory phenomena in the capillaries and venules which contributes to the development of small blood vessel disease.

Platelet Proteins

By analogy to Spiro's work in the renal glomerulus, Waitzman has recently studied the glucosyltransferase activity of platelets obtained from diabetic subjects and has found it to be markedly elevated (Waitzman, Colley, and Mardelli-Olkoska, 1977). Since this enzyme is thought to be related to the facilitation of platelet adhesion to the exposed collagen of damaged vascular endothelium, such an increase in its activity could be related not only to the increased platelet adhesiveness, but also to the increased incidence of microthromboses and large blood vessel disease in the diabetic subject (Colwell, Chambers, and Laimins, 1975). The relationship between abnormal glycosylation of platelet proteins and the functional abnormalities of diabetic platelets is currently under active investigation in the laboratories of Dr. Charles Peterson at Rockefeller University.

Hemoglobin

Another hematological abnormality which results from the spontaneous nonenzymatic addition of glucose molecules to proteins is the abnormally elevated percentage of hemoglobin A_{I_c} in the erythrocytes of poorly controlled diabetic subjects. When hemoglobin A is exposed to glucose, the amino group of the amino-terminal valine of the *beta* chain can form a Schiff-base linkage with the aldehyde group of the glucose molecule. Subsequently, *via* an Amadori rearrangement, the glucose molecule becomes covalently and irreversibly bound to hemoglobin (Bunn, Haney, Gabbay, and Gallop, 1975). Since the formation of hemoglobin A_{I_c} is a nonenzymatic process, the proportion of erythrocyte hemoglobin which is glycosylated at any given time provides a rough estimate of the glucose concentration to which the erythrocyte has been exposed over the preceding several months and, thus, can be used as a rough monitor of the degree of diabetic control. However, although elevated levels of hemoglobin A_{I_c} may be useful to the physician in the assessment of patient compliance, it may have pathological consequences for the patient himself. Similar to hemoblogin F, hemoglobin AI_c discharges oxygen to the tissues less readily than does normal hemoglobin and is less sensitive to the allosteric effects of red cell 2,3-diphosphoglyceric acid (2,3-DPG)(Gandhi and Bleicher, 1975). Since the poorly controlled diabetic has decreased erythrocyte 2,3-DPG concentrations as well, this combination may seriously impair his ability to oxygenate his tissues and, consequently, may contribute to the development of large blood vessel disease. Furthermore, since 2,3-DPG interferes with the formation of glycosylated hemoglobins, a decrease in the concentration of this compound in the red cell may accelerate the rate of hemoglobin AI_c synthesis under conditions of extremely poor diabetic control (Stevens, Vlassara, Abati, and Cerami, 1977).

Other hematologic abnormalities which are postulated to be directly related to hyperglycemia through abnormal glycosylation of peptides include the previously discussed abnormality in platelet function and decreased leukocyte adherance to a glass-wool column (Peterson, Jones, Koenig, Melvin, and Lehrman, 1977). Obviously, these biochemical derangements may be directly related to virtually all of the complications of the diabetic state and will, undoubtedly, be the focus of intense research activity over the next few years.

POLYOL PATHWAY

Lens

Speculation that increased activity of the polyol pathway could be related to the development of complications in various tissues of the diabetic stemmed from early studies of "sugar" cataracts in experimental animals (van Heyningen, 1959). Van Heyningen demonstrated that the enzymes of the polyol pathway (aldose reductase and sorbitol dehydrogenase) are present in the rat lens and that the induction of alloxan-diabetes results in increased concentrations of sorbitol in this tissue. She proposed that the accumulation of sorbitol within the lens might offer an explanation for the development of cataracts in animals with experimental diabetes. Further evidence for the participation of increased polyol pathway activity in the pathogenesis of cataracts has been provided by *in vitro* studies (Kinoshita, 1965). When the lens of the rabbit is incubated in the presence of high glucose concentrations, the observed increase in sorbitol content is paralleled by an increase in the water content of this tissue. Since polyols are known to cross certain cell membranes slowly, Kinoshita proposed that the accumulation of polyols within the lens could lead to tissue damage as a result of their osmotic activity. In support of this theory was his observation that by simply increasing the osmolality of the incubation medium, he could prevent the accumulation of water by and the eventual development of cataract in the incubated lens. Further experimental evidence for the direct participation of the polyol pathway in "sugar" cataracts is provided by the observations that inhibition of aldose reductase activity prevents the formation of cataracts (Chylack and Kinoshita, 1969) and animals whose lenses lack aldose reductase do not develop cataracts when they are rendered diabetic (Kuck, 1970).

That the development of "sugar" cataracts is due exclusively to intracellular osmotic phenomena is probably an oversimplification. Workers in St. Louis have observed a lack of parallelism between the polyol and water content of the lenses of galactose-fed rats (Stewart, Kurien, Sherman, and Cotlier, 1968). In addition, electron microscopic studies of the developing "sugar" cataract have demonstrated that the earliest morphologic alterations are those of cellular proliferation, an increase in the amount of endoplasmic reticulum and intercellular fluid accumulation rather than a simple increase in the intracellular water content of the lens. It is possible that these discrepancies have a biochemical explanation, since exposure of the lens to increased ambient glucose concentrations produces numerous biochemical alterations in addition to the increase in polyol pathway activity (Chylack and Kinoshita, 1969). An elevated glucose concentration decreases the ability of the lens to maintain normal concentrations of reduced glutathione, ATP, myoinositol, sodium, and potassium. The reduction in reduced glutathione may be due to competition for NADPH by the increase in polyol pathway activity and may reduce the capacity of this tissue to respond to oxidant stress. The reduction in ATP may limit the availability of energy required for the maintenance of normal intracellular sodium and water concentrations. The inability of the lens to maintain normal intracellular myoinositol concentrations may decrease the capacity of this tissue to synthesize phosphoinositides, a process which is thought to be related to ion transport (Hendrickson and Reinertsen, 1971).

Thus, the lens has served as an excellent model in which to study the mechanisms by which the biochemical alterations secondary to exposure to elevated glucose concentrations may lead to pathological changes. While it is fairly well established that increased polyol pathway activity is involved in the pathogenesis of "sugar" cataracts, it is becoming equally clear that a number of other (and possibly unrelated) biochemical alterations could play supporting roles in this process.

Nerve

By analogy to the lens, increased polyol pathway activity has been speculated to play a role in the structural and functional abnormalities in the peripheral nerve which are almost universal concomitants of diabetes mellitus in both animals and man. The presence of the polyol pathway in peripheral nerve has been unequivocally established (Gabbay, Merola, and Field, 1966) and its activity appears to be exquisitely sensitive to the ambient glucose concentration (Stewart, Sherman, Kurien, Moonsammy, and Wisgerhof, 1967). Since the product of the polyol pathway (fructose) has been found to increase in the distal segment of the transected nerve at a time when the Schwann cells are proliferating, it has been speculated that such localization could account, in part, for the segmental demyelination associated with diabetic neuropathy, since the Schwann cell is responsible for the elaboration of myelin.

The induction of experimental diabetes consistently leads to elevated concentrations of polyol pathway intermediates, as well as decreased myoinositol concentrations and decreased nerve conduction velocities in the sciatic nerve of the rat (Gabbay, 1973; Greene, De Jesus, and Winegrad, 1975). In these experiments, careful insulin therapy was found to correct all of these abnormalities. Of particular interest, however, was the observation that only when complete normalization of the fluctuations in blood glucose concentrations were achieved could the functional abnormality be corrected.

In contrast to the observations in the lens, no increase in the water content of the peripheral nerve of the diabetic rat can be detected. Similar to the lens, the water content of the nerve does not appear to parallel the polyol content in galactose-fed rats (Stewart *et al.*, 1968). Thus, there is, at present, no evidence to suggest that osmotic phenomena resulting from increased polyol pathway activity are involved in the structural or functional abnormalities observed in diabetic neuropathy. That increased polyol pathway activity *per se* may be related to neuropathy is suggested, however, by the studies in progress to evaluate the effect of inhibitors of aldose reductase upon the course of diabetic neuropathy (Gabbay, personal communication). On the other hand, the observations of Greene *et al.* that the decreased motor nerve conduction velocity could be corrected by oral myoinositol supplementation (a maneuver which had no effect upon the nerve concentrations of glucose or polyol pathway intermediates) suggests that increased polyol pathway activity in the peripheral nerve of the diabetic may be an epiphenomenon which is not directly related to the pathogenesis of diabetic neuropathy (Greene *et al.*, 1975).

Aorta

Studies of the distribution of the enzyme, aldose reductase, have revealed that the polyol pathway is widely distributed in mammalian tissues (Clements, Weaver, and Winegrad, 1969). Among those tissues in which this enzyme has been demonstrated is included the media of the arterial wall, a primary target tissue for the complications of diabetes (Clements, Morrison, and Winegrad, 1969). The rabbit thoracic aortic media has been found to contain concentrations of sorbitol which are significantly higher than those of the rabbit plasma (Morrison, Clements, and Winegrad, 1973) and which increase still further when the aorta is incubated with elevated glucose concentrations. Similar to the lens, this increase in the sorbitol concentration is accompanied by an increase in the water content of the aorta which appears to decrease oxygen diffusion and to increase the rate of lactate production by this tissue. That the increase in water content is due to increased polyol pathway activity is suggested by the observation that inhibition of aldose reductase will prevent the development of this abnormality. However, the accumulation of polyol pathway intermediates in the aorta is minuscule compared to that observed in the lens, and cannot account for the increase in water content on an osmotic basis. In addition, since elevation of the ambient myoinositol concentration has been found to prevent the increase in water content, the decrease in oxygen uptake, and the increase in lactate formation, it is possible that alterations in myoinositol metabolism may be of more importance than increased polyol pathway activity in the pathogenesis of these derangements.

ABNORMAL MYOINOSITOL METABOLISM

Myoinositol Metabolism in the Human with Diabetes Mellitus

A recurrent theme which runs through the speculations concerning the relationship between the polyol pathway and diabetic complications is that increased activity of this pathway in all tissues which have been adequately studied is always accompanied by derangements in the metabolism of myoinositol. Myoinositol is an hexahydroxy derivative of cyclohexane which has been found to be present in significant concentrations in all mammalian organs. Although its physiologic functions have not been clearly established, the incorporation of myoinositol into membrane phospholipids has been thought to be related to numerous cellular processes including electrolyte (Hendrickson and Reinertsen, 1971) and amino acid transport (Lembach and Charalampous, 1967), nerve impulse transmission (Pumphrey, 1969), and the stimulated secretion of various intracellular peptides (Clements and Rhoten, 1976; Michell, 1975). It would be anticipated, therefore, that impairment of either the intracellular transport of myoinositol or of its rate of incorporation into phospholipids would result in pathological changes in the affected tissues. Since the active intracellular transport of myoinositol is inhibited by elevated glucose concentrations (Caspary and Crane, 1970), it is not surprising that the intracellular content of this material is decreased in the lens and nerve of animals with experimental diabetes. Furthermore, the competitive nature of the inhibition of myoinositol transport by glucose would explain the observation of Greene *et al.* that the decreased nerve myoinositol content of the diabetic rat nerve could be normalized by diet-induced elevation of the plasma myoinositol concentration (Greene *et al.*, 1975). The possibility that the mechanism by which this manipulation resulted in normalization of nerve conduction velocities was related to the provision of adequate amounts of substrate for the formation of phosphoinositides has not been studied. However, it should be point out that, despite the apparent reciprocal relationship between polyol pathway activity and intracellular myoinositol concentrations, these two phenomena are unrelated manifestations of the effects of hyperglycemia upon certain tissues. Increased polyol pathway activity results from increased intracellular concentrations of glucose in those cells which contain the enzymes of the polyol pathway, whereas the decrease in myoinositol concentrations results from the combined effects of extracellular glucose upon intracellular myoinositol transport and of intracellular glucose upon its efflux.

The salutary effect of dietary myoinositol supplementation upon the functional neurologic abnormalities in the diabetic rat prompted us to study myoinositol metabolism in human subjects with diabetes mellitus (Clements and Reynertson, 1977). As had been previously observed, we noted that the urinary excretion of myoinositol was markedly increased in the diabetic and accounted for roughly one-third of his daily dietary myoinositol intake. Despite this fact, the mean plasma myoinositol concentration in a large group of diabetics was significantly elevated. This observation can be accounted for by the increased incidence of functional renal abnormalities in the diabetics since the plasma myoinositol concentration is positively correlated with the serum urea nitrogen and creatinine concentrations. In uncontrolled diabetics with normal renal function, the fasting plasma myoinositol concentrations were normal, but rose to pathologically elevated levels following the oral ingestion of myoinositol. The possibilities that this abnormal rise in plasma myoinositol concentration was due to either abnormally rapid rates of gastrointestinal absorption, to decreased rates of myoinositol disappearance from the plasma, or to normal rates of absorption into a decreased myoinositol pool, were studied by radioactive techniques. In six poorly controlled diabetics, the disappearance rate of myoinositol was found to be similar to that of the controls. However, their myoinositol pool size was decreased to less than half of that observed in the nondiabetics. Following the institution of careful insulin therapy, oral myoinositol tolerance and the myoinositol pool size returned to normal. In the untreated diabetic, the myoinositol pool size approximated the extracellular fluid space, whereas in the control subjects and in the treated diabetics, it was found to be roughly twice the size of the extracellular fluid compartment. Therefore, these data are consistent with *in vitro* studies and suggest that uncontrolled hyperglycemia may impair the intracellular transport of myoinositol in the human diabetic.

To determine whether the plasma myoinositol concentration and fractional retention of ingested myoinositol could be influenced by the amount of myoinositol in the diet, we developed diets which provided either low (~ 200 mg), normal (~ 600 mg), or high (~ 2500 mg) daily myoinositol intakes. In preliminary studies, we have observed that in diabetics the mean plasma myoinositol concentration varied as a function of the amount of the myoinositol in the diet, whereas in nondiabetics it did not. In addition, the fractional excretion of myoinositol in the urine could be profoundly decreased by increasing the dietary myoinositol intake. Although direct analyses of tissue myoinositol content have not been performed, these data suggest that increased dietary myoinositol intake may elevate the plasma myoinositol concentration and, in part, overcome the defect in intracellular myoinositol transport in the human diabetic.

Nerve Myoinositol Metabolism

To determine whether increased myoinositol intake could influence nerve function in diabetic neuropathy, we have carried out sequential electrophysiological studies of patients with clinically apparent neuropathy prior to and for periods of up to six months on high myoinositol diets. As indicated in Figure 1, increases in the median motor and sural sensory nerve conduction velocities were observed in the first three patients studied. Subsequently, in a larger group of ten patients, we have observed statistically significant increases in the median motor, peroneal motor, and sural sensory nerve conduction velocities as indicated in Table 1. In all but one subject, these increases were accompanied by subjective improvement in the symptoms of neuropathy. In contrast, little objective improvement could be detected by physical examination. Obviously, a group of patients with established diabetic neuropathy is not the ideal population in which to evaluate the effects of increased myoinositol intake, since one would expect that their defective nerve function would be, to a large extent, irreversible. Studies of the influence of dietary myoinositol upon nerve function in diabetic patients without clinical evidence of diabetic neuropathy will be required, since the magnitude of an effect (if any) should be greater in such patients.

To determine whether the effect of hyperglycemia upon nerve myoinositol metabolism is due to impaired intracellular myoinositol transport or to decreased rates of incorporation of myoinositol into nerve phosphoinositides, we have studied these phenomena in

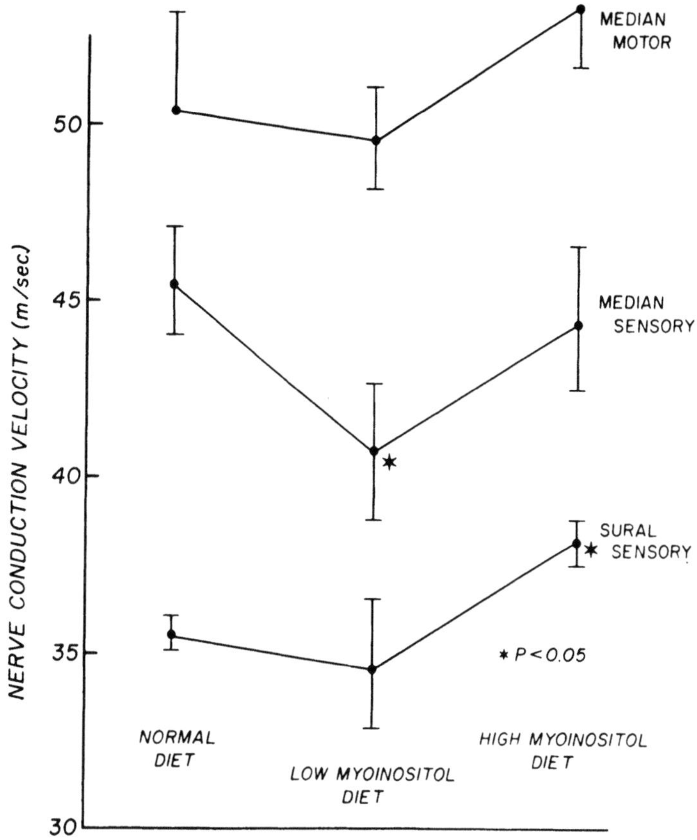

Figure 1. *Mean nerve conduction velocities in three patients with diabetic neuropathy during sequential two-week periods of ingestion of normal, low, and high myoinositol diets.*

Table 1. *NERVE CONDUCTION VELOCITIES (M/Sec) IN TEN PATIENTS WITH DIABETIC NEUROPATHY BEFORE AND DURING THE INGESTION OF HIGH MYOINOSITOL DIETS FOR PERIODS UP TO SIX MONTHS*

Nerve studied	Control Diet	High myoinositol diet	p of paired differences
Median motor	47.9 ± 1.2	51.4 ± 0.9	< 0.005
Median sensory	38.1 ± 2.0	37.9 ± 1.3	n.s.
Peroneal motor	39.3 ± 2.1	40.0 ± 1.7	< 0.05
Sural Sensory	32.1 ± 2.3	37.6 ± 1.1	< 0.01

the rat nerve. Age-matched controls and rats with streptozotocin-diabetes of 14-days duration were injected intraperitoneally with 50 μCi of 2-^{3}H-myoinositol and their sciatic nerves were excised after four hours. The water-soluble, myoinositol-derived radioactivity was determined in nerve homogenates and the incorporation of myoinositol into phospholipids was determined in chloroform: methanol extracts. As shown in Figure 2, we observed a 20% decrease in the recovery of 2-^{3}H-myoinositol-derived water-soluble radioactivity from the diabetic rat nerves. Although this decrease is not statistically significant, it may indicate that the transport of myoinositol into the nerve is decreased in the diabetic animals. In contrast, a marked decrease in the recovery of lipid-bound 2-^{3}H-myoinositol was observed. Whether this decrease in incorporation of radioactivity into phospholipids is due to limited substrate availability or to alterations in the nerve CDP-diglyceride:inositol transferase activity must await direct enzymatic analysis. Since the Km of CDP-diglyceride:inositol transferase is extraordinarily high, it is possible that rather slight decreases in the neural myoinositol concentrations could have a profound influence upon the rate of phosphatidylinositol synthesis (Takenawa and Egawa, 1977). In any case, these data suggest that hyperglycemia results in a profound alteration in the phosphoinositide metabolism of the peripheral nerve and raise the possibility

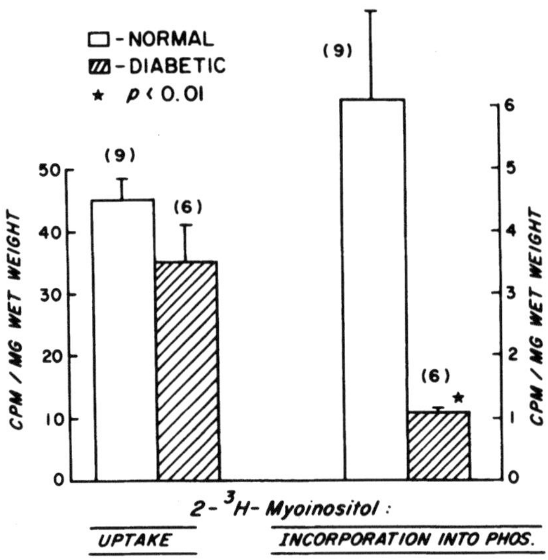

Figure 2. Recovery of water-soluble myoinositol-derived radioactivity (uptake) and lipid-bound 2-^{3}H-myoinositol (incorporation into phospholipids) from the sciatic nerves of nondiabetic and streptozotocin-diabetic rats four hours following the intraperitoneal injection of 2-^{3}H-myoinositol (50 μCi).

that this metabolic alteration could be related to the reversible functional abnormalities in the diabetic rat nerve.

SUMMARY AND CONCLUSIONS

During the past few years, remarkable strides have been made in the elucidation of biochemical mechanisms which could play a role in the pathogenesis of diabetic complications. In this discussion, only a few of these mechanisms have been considered--abnormal protein glycosylation, increased polyol pathway activity, and disturbed myoinositol metabolism. Since the biochemical abnormalities which result from insulin deficiency and hyperglycemia are legion, it may be presumptuous to have singled out only three of these abnormalities for consideration. At the present time, however, the possible relationship between these biochemical derangements and diabetic complications have received the most study. It should be pointed out that these studies have not established an unequivocal relationship between any of these mechanisms and pathological changes in any tissue. Undoubtedly, in the next few years, a number of other potentially toxic biochemical mechanisms will be discovered and will receive extensive study. It is probably safe to speculate that the development of a specific complication in any given tissue of the diabetic results from a complex interaction of biochemical, genetic, and local tissue factors. Nonetheless, the demonstration of potentially damaging biochemical mechanisms which are activated by hyperglycemia in certain target tissues of the diabetic raises the possibility that abnormal fluctuations in the blood glucose concentration could actively contribute to the pathological changes in those tissues.

REFERENCES

Beisswenger, P.J. 1976. Glomerular basement membrane: Biosynthesis and chemical composition in the streptozotocin diabetic rat. *J. Clin. Invest.* **58**:844-852.

Beisswenger, P.J. and Spiro, R.G. 1970. Human glomerular basement membrane: Chemical alteration in diabetes mellitus. *Science* **168**:596-598.

Bunn, H.F., Haney, D.N., Gabbay, K.H., and Gallop, P.M. 1975. Further identification of the nature and linkage of the carbohydrate in hemoglobin A_{Ic}. *Biochem. Biophys. Res. Commun.* **67**:103-109.

Caspary, W.F. and Crane, R.K. 1970. Active transport of myoinositol and its relation to the sugar transport system in hamster small intestine. *Biochim. Biophys. Acta* **203**:308-316.

Chylack, L.T. Jr. and Kinoshita, J.H. 1969. A biochemical evaluation of a cataract induced in a high glucose medium. *Invest. Ophthal.* **8**:401-412.

Clements, R.S. Jr., Morrison, A.D., and Winegrad, A.I. 1969.

Polyol pathway in aorta: Regulation by hormones. *Science* **166**:1007-1008.

Clements, R.S. Jr. and Reynertson, R. 1977. Myoinositol metabolism in diabetes mellitus: Effect of insulin treatment. *Diabetes* **26**:215-221.

Clements, R.S. Jr. and Rhoten, W.B. 1976. Phosphoinositide metabolism and insulin secretion from isolated rat pancreatic islets. *J. Clin. Invest.* **57**:684-691.

Clements, R.S. Jr., Weaver, J.P., and Winegrad, A.I. 1969. The distribution of polyol:NADP oxidoreductase in mammalian tissues. *Biochem. Biophys. Res. Commun.* **37**:347-353.

Cohen, M.P. and Vogt, C. 1972. Evidence for enchanced basement membrane synthesis and lysine hydroxylation in renal glomerulus in experimental diabetes. *Biochem. Biophys. Res. Commun.* **49**:1542-1546.

Colwell, J.A., Chambers, A., and Laimins, M. 1975. Inhibition of labile aggregation-stimulating substance (LASS) and platelet aggregation in diabetes mellitus. *Diabetes* **24**:684-687.

Fushimi, H. and Tarui, S. 1976. β-glycosidases and diabetic microangiopathy. I. Decreases of β-glycosidase activities in diabetic rat kidney. *J. Biochem.* **79**:265-270.

Gabbay, K.H. 1973. pp 417-424. IN R.A. Camerini-Davalos and H.S. Cole (Eds.) *Vascular and neurologic changes in early diabetes.* New York: Academic Press.

Gabbay, K.H., Merola, L.O., and Field, R.A. 1966. Sorbitol pathway: Presence in nerve and cord with substrate accumulation in diabetes. *Science* **151**:209-210.

Gandhi, V.S. and Bleicher, S.J. 1975. "Fast" hemoglobin, diabetes and pregnancy. *Diabetes* **24**:415.

Grant, M.E., Kefalides, N.A., and Prockop, D.J. 1972. The biosynthesis of basement membrane collagen in embryonic chick cells and a time-dependent conversion to chains in intact lens. *J. Biol. Chem.* **247**:3545-3551.

Greene, D.A., De Jesus, P.V., and Winegrad, A.I. 1975. Effects of insulin and dietary myoinositol on impaired peripheral motor nerve conduction velocity in acute streptozotocin diabetes. *J. Clin. Invest.* **55**:1326-1336.

Hendrickson, H.S. and Reinertsen, J.L. 1971. Phosphoinositide interconversion: A model for control of Na^+ and K^+ permeability in the nerve axon membrane. *Biochem. Biophys. Res. Commun.* **44**:1258-1264.

Kefalides, N.A. 1974. Biochemical properties of human glomerular basement membrane in normal and diabetic kidneys. *J. Clin. Invest.* **53**:403-407.

Khalifa, A.S. and Cohen, M.P. 1975. Glomerular protocollagen lysylhydroxylase activity in streptozotocin diabetes. *Biochim. Biophys. Acta* **386**:332-339.

Kinoshita, J.H. 1965. Cataracts in galactosemia. *Invest. Ophthal.* **4**:786-799.

Kuck, J.F.R. Jr. 1970. Response of the mouse lens to high concentrations of glucose or galactose. *Ophthal. Res.* **1**:166-174.
Lemback, K. and Charalampous, F.C. 1967. Metabolic functions of myoinositol. VI. Impairment of amino acid transport in KB cells caused by inositol deficiency. *J. Biol. Chem.* **242**: 2606-2614.
McMillan, D.E. 1972. Elevation of glycoprotein fucose in diabetes mellitus. *Diabetes* **21**:863-871.
Michell, R.H. 1975. Inositol phospholipids and cell surface receptor function. *Biochim. Biophys. Acta* **415**:81-147.
Morrison, A.D., Clements, R.S. Jr., and Winegrad, A.I. 1973. Effects of elevated glucose concentrations on the metabolism of the aortic wall. *J. Clin. Invest.* **51**:3114-3123.
Peterson, C.M., Jones, R.L., Koenig, R.J., Melvin, E.T., and Lehrman, M.L. 1977. Reversible hematologic sequelae of diabetes mellitus. *Ann. Int. Med.* **86**:425-429.
Pumphrey, A.M. 1969. Incorporation of (^{32}P) orthophosphate into brain-slice phospholipids and their precursors: Effects of electrical stimulation. *Biochem. J.* **112**:61-70.
Stewart, M.A., Kurien, M.M., Sherman, W.R., and Cotlier, E.V. 1968. Inositol changes in nerve and lens of galactose fed rats. *J. Neurochem.* **15**:941-946.
Stewart, M.A., Sherman, W.R., Kurien, M.M., Moonsammy, G.I., and Wisgerhof, M. 1967. Polyol accumulations in nervous tissue of rats with experimental diabetes and galactosemia. *J. Neurochem.* **14**:1057-1066.
Stevens, V.J., Vlassara, H., Abati, A., and Cerami, A. 1977. Nonenzymatic glycosylation of hemoglobin. *J. Biol. Chem.* **252**: 2998-3002.
Takenawa, T. and Egawa, K. 1977. CDP-diglyceride:inositol transferase from rat liver. *J. Biol. Chem.* **252**:5419-5423.
van Heyningen, R. 1959. Formation of polyols by the lens of the rat with "sugar" cataract. *Nature* **184**:194-195.
Wahl, P., Deppermann, D., Deschner, W., Fuchs, E., and Rexroth, W. 1973. pp. 147-153. IN R.A. Camerini-Davolos and H.S. Cole (Eds.) *Vascular and neurologic changes in early diabetes.* New York: Academic Press.
Waitzman, M.B., Colley, A.M., and Nardelli-Olkoska, K. 1977. Metabolic approaches to studies on diabetic microangiopathy. *Diabetes* **26**:510-517.
Westberg, N.G. and Michael, A.F. 1973. Human glomerular basement membrane: Chemical composition in diabetes mellitus. *Acta Med. Scand.* **144**:39-47.

DISCUSSION FOLLOWING DR. CLEMENTS' TALK

Dr. Werner

I should have prefaced Dr. Clements' remarks with the extreme importance of this kind of work. It is obvious to most people that relatively few people die these days from the complications of ketoacidosis and coma, but the high incidence of morbidity and mortality obviously is due to the tissue complications of the diabetes. These facts make it so imperative that a way is found to stop these complications and Dr. Clements' work is foremost in the area of these studies.

Dr. Brownlee

I think that myoinositol is an extremely exciting area. I want to ask you two questions about the last slide that you showed concerning incorporation of myoinositol into the phospholipids.

The first question is, was the dose of labeled myoinositol calculated on a weight basis or was it an identical amount of radioactivity injected into the diabetic and normal animals? The reason I'm asking that is because the diabetics weigh less than the normal.

The second question is, was this data corrected for pool size? You have shown that the myoinositol pool size is different in the diabetic subjects as well as the fact that the levels in the plasma were increased in the diabetic following an oral load. If the specific activity of the myoinositol that you injected was diluted to a different degree in the diabetic than in the normal, then the incorporation data, rather than simply reflecting rates of incorporation, could also reflect relative degrees of dilution by plasma myoinositol.

Dr. Clements

Those are very pertinent questions. The amount of radioactivity which we administered was constant from animal to animal. We measured the specific activity of the plasma myoinositol pool throughout as well as the conversion of tritiated myoinositol to tritiated water. We were unable to determine any differences in the specific activity of the circulating plasma myoinositol in these animals.

One other point which your question raises is that if there were to be a slight increase in the water content of the nerve of the diabetic rat, then one could get an increase in the ratio of the free myoinositol concentration relative to the radioactivity within the nerve pool which would, in part, account for the decreased specific activity of myoinositol in this tissue. I can't say, at the present time, that there is a significant difference in the pool size of the diabetic versus the nondiabetic rat because we have not finished the analysis of the pool size and half time of myoinositol disappearance in these animals. For such analyses, it would have been preferable if we had given the radioactivity intravenously. However, as yet we don't have any good evidence that there is a difference in the plasma myoinositol specific activity in the two groups of animals.

Dr. Levine

May I ask, Dr. Clements, whether you consider myoinositol an essential nutrient?

Dr. Clements

Dr. Levine, I appreciate your question, but I cannot consider it to be an essential nutrient, since the FDA ruled two years ago that it is not. However, prior to that time it had been considered to be an essential nutrient.

Dr. Levine

What is its biochemical origin?

Dr. Clements

Biochemically, it is the result of a cyclization of a glucose-6-phosphate molecule with subsequent dephosphorylation and reduction.

Dr. Levine

In the plant kingdom?

Dr. Clements

The members of the plant kingdom are quite capable of synthesizing myoinositol. Numerous mammalian organs, outstanding among which are the testicles, also can convert glucose-6-phosphate to inositol. The concentration of myoinositol in boar semen is roughly 2000 mg/dℓ whereas in human semen it is only 200 mg/dℓ.

Dr. Levine

If you'll permit me, I'll tell you a story. Years ago at a conference I asked the expert on semen and seminal fluids, Thaddeus Mann from Cambridge, as to why there is fructose in semen.

He thought awhile and said that they use fructose for locomotion, so to speak, and the reason for that, it seems to him, is that finding themselves in territory where they would have to compete for glucose with an enormous number of epithelial uterine cells, they develop the need for a substrate which the epithelial cells of the uterus could not participate in. It's an excellent evolutionary dodge.

Is myoinositol similar? Do they use it for anything?

Dr. Clements

They don't appear to use it for anything that we know of. It is present in very high concentrations in seeds and in most processes involving germination.

I am aware of Dr. Mann's speculation as to the fact that the spermatozoa utilize fructose as their preferred substrate. However, a major problem with that speculation is that the stallion has a low seminal fluid fructose concentration which does not appear to interfere with the function of his spermatozoa.

Dr. Levine

The older literature described a very large concentration of inositol in cardiac muscle. This begins to have a kind of interest closer to home for the diabetic. Would cardiac myoinositol in the ordinary diabetic population be decreased? Is that of any importance from the standpoint of myocardial metabolism and myocarcial survival?

Dr. Clements

You are aware, I think, of the studies of Dr. Gerald Levy on effects of histamine stimulation of cardiac action on the rates of incorporation of myoinositol into the membrane phospholipids of the myocardium. Myoinositol got its prefix from the fact that it was first isolated from mammalian muscle. Its physiologic function in muscle is not known to the present day, nor is it known whether muscle actively transports this material. It must be transported because its concentration in muscle is considerably higher than that of plasma. Why it is necessary for particular organs to actively concentrate this material or the particular membrane functions which it serves in these tissues is not known. Nor is it known whether the diabetic has a decrease in muscle levels of this material or in the rate of its incorporation into the muscle phospholipids. I think those might be very crucial questions to be approached in the future.

Dr. Vorbeck

I would like to comment with regard to studies on basement membrane biosynthesis. Dr. Grant Schmidt, working in our laboratory with animals that were spontaneously diabetic, was able to demonstrate rather significant increases in basement membrane glucosyl transferase in the preparations from the kidney cortex (Schmidt, Martin, Townsend, and Vorbeck, 1977). Indeed, in this same group of animals Dr. Jim Esterly, in our department, was also able to demonstrate rather significant increases in the thickening of skeletal muscle basement membrane of diabetic animals. So the biochemical data correlated very nicely with the ultrastructural studies in this particular animal model.

Dr. Clements

Dr. Beisswenger's model was a little bit different, in that he was studying both short- and long-term streptozotocin diabetic rats. Up to a period of 14 months he could see no morphologic changes in the glomeruli. Dr. Beisswenger is not an electron microscopist, so it is possible that he might have missed some subtle abnormalities in their basement membranes.

Dr. Vorbeck

These were spontaneously diabetic animals in the 20- to 22-month age range. The normal life span of the animals was somewhere around four to five years.

Dr. Clements

The animals you describe had extremely long-term diabetes and there may be a significant difference between the chemically-induced and the spontaneous forms of diabetes with regard to the rate of progression of these lesions in rodent models.

Dr. Werner

Dr. Clements, concerning the myoinositol tolerance test, do you know which tissues are responsible for picking up the myoinositol? Are they noninsulin-responsive tissues?

Dr. Clements

We don't know. Virtually every mammalian tissue has intracellular myoinositol concentrations which are orders of magnitude higher than those of plasma. Perhaps as endocrinologists we can be proud of the fact that the endocrine tissues maintain the highest concentrations and the nerves come second. The pituitary, the adrenal, and the thyroid have extraordinarily high concentrations, but the only normal mammalian tissues which are known to actively transport myoinositol are the kidney, the ileum, and the lens. So far the transport mechanisms in other tissues have not been studied. In the pancreatic islet we have found no evidence for active transport nor has Dr. Lacy's group. We do know that the concentration of myoinositol is approximately one *millimolar* in the pancreatic islet, so with appropriate techniques we should be able to demonstrate either active transport or endogenous synthesis of myoinositol in this tissue.

Dr. Werner

What about glycosylation of other proteins besides structural proteins? For example, of enzymes leading to alterations in activity or degradation? Is there any information in this area?

Dr. Clements

There is very little that I'm aware of. There are a number of workers, including Oscar Touster, who are actively involved in the analysis of the explanation for the abnormal levels of the glycohydrolases in the plasma and urine of the diabetic patients, but to my knowledge their direct role in the breakdown of such glycoproteins has not been clarified.

Maybe Dr. Peterson would like to comment on that because he's actively working on this problem.

Dr. Peterson

We don't know anything about enzymes and we haven't really looked at them: I can clarify some of the things on structural proteins that we have looked at, and I guess the key word is rate. When hemoglobin is glycosylated, it is analogous to carbamylated protein in that its rate of oxidation is greatly increased. This, also, appears to be what is happening with α-crystalline in the lens (Cerami, Koenig, Peterson, and Stevens, 1978). If one glycosylates α-crystalline or if α-crystalline is taken from diabetic animals and kept under nitrogen, it will stay fairly clear. If it is exposed to oxygen, it does turn cloudy.

If our hypothesis, in terms of glycosylations applies to the lens, it would appear that what is happening is that the rate of oxidation of the lens protein is altered folowing glycosylation reactions.

It is also interesting to compare the lens anatomy of what we observed *in vitro* with glucose as opposed to galactose, where you get actually a swelling of the lens. With glucose you get some swelling but you also get at the suture line the very distinct beginning opacification which is more analogous to what you see in diabetics--that posterior subcapsular edema progressing to actual punctate sclerosis.

Dr. Clements

Could your observations concerning the α-crystalline be directly affected by the decreased levels of reduced glutathione in the lens of the diabetic animals analogous to the decreased levels of reduced glutathione in the erythrocyte?

Dr. Peterson

Yes. The problem with all this is, where is "Sutton's Law?" That is, "where is the money;" which is the major pathological entity? And I can't say that any more than you can.

The other thing I could say about the erythrocyte is that the data with 2,3-DPG is a little bit conflicting. We found that most of the phosphorylated glycolytic intermediates in diabetic red cells that we evaluated were elevated except for 2,3-DPG. Glycolytic intermediates with a phosphate and an aldehyde or ketone are competitive inhibitors for the n-terminal site (Stevens, Vlassara, Abati, and Cerami, 1977).

Dr. Clements

I think we can safely say that the development of complications in any tissue is going to be a composite of the interactions of genetic, biochemical, hormonal, humoral, and local tissue factors.

Dr. Levine

Again, coming back to myoinositol, are you aware of any experiments in a mammalian species deliberately fed a diet free of myoinositol? What happens to such mammalian species and its functions?

Dr. Clements

Yes, Needham studied this question in the 30's. In the rat it leads to speckled eye disease, which is a depigmentation developing around the eyes and loss of hair. Unfortunately, in retrospect, Needham was giving a myoinositol-deficient diet but not a myoinositol-free diet. In addition, studies which we have carried out with Dr. Diethelm have shown that the human kidney is capable of making two to three *grams* of myoinositol per day under normal circumstances. Needham found that he could keep his rats on myoinositol-free diets for months and yet their carcass myoinositol concentration did not change at all over that period of time.

The reason for thinking that this material might be a vitamin comes from Eagle's original studies of tissue culture requirements in which all human cells, and most other mammalian cells, absolutely required myoinositol for growth and division *in vitro*. Since myoinositol was an essential requirement for human cells in tissue culture, it was speculated to be a dietary requirement. This possibility has not been reevaluated.

Dr. Heimberg

A few years ago there was discussion that the conversion of the triphosphoinositides and diphosphoinositides was involved in some way in the nerve impulse, presumably involving a change in calcium transport and differences in calcium solubility of the di/triphosphoinositides. Is there any change, to your knowledge, in this reaction or conversion in diabetes, or in experimental diabetes?

Dr. Clements

We haven't seen any difference in the ratio of di- and triphosphoinositides in the peripheral nerve of the diabetic animal. The speculation concerning the effects of chelation of calcium by the di- and triphosphoinositides is based on the fact that, when you stimulate a peripheral nerve electrically, there is a marked increase in the rate of turnover or incorporation of radioactive myoinositol into these phosphoinositides. Triphosphoinositide is an extremely good chelator of calcium ions while diphosphoinositide has a somewhat lesser affinity. Monophosphatidylinositol has a still lower affinity, but will weakly chelate calcium. Hendrickson and Reynertson originally speculated that the turnover of di- and triphosphatidylinositol might be related to calcium fluxes or the freeing up of cytosolic calcium which plays a role in nerve impulse conduction. To my knowledge, there is no evidence for abnormalities of the ratios of these two in the diabetic nerve.

However, I can say with some assurance that, if one exposes phosphatidylinositol micelles to calcium concentrations which are in the physiologic range, one observes marked inhibition of the lipid phase transition characteristics of those micelles. In fact, one will get total abolition of gel- to liquid-crystalline phase transition at calcium concentrations above one *millimolar*. This phenomenon is only observed when the calcium is within the micelle. Calcium external to the micelle will not cause the inhibition of phase transition.

Dr. Heimberg

There was also, I believe, a difference in sodium solubility with the mono-, di-, and triphosphoinositides?

Dr. Clements

Yes. I don't think that the experimental proof of that was rigorous, but this was the speculation of Hendrickson and Reynertson.

Dr. Williamson

It's my understanding that the beneficial effects of myoinositol on motor nerve conduction velocity are not observed if you give excess amounts of myoinositol. I wonder if you could comment on problems of toxicity.

Dr. Clements

Tnat is quite true. In Green's and Winegrad's studies they observed that if they fed diabetic animals 1% myoinositol (by weight) that there was marked improvement in nerve function. However, if they increased the dietary myoinositol content to 3%, they observed deterioration in nerve conduction velocities.

In our previous studies we had observed that feeding 35% myoinositol to rats profoundly decreased their nerve conduction velocities. What the mechanism is, is a completely open question. The mechanism which I would like to propose is that in diabetes the decreased plasma myoinositol concentrations or decreased rates of transport of myoinositol into the target tissues could impair the rates of phosphoinositide synthesis. In contrast, markedly elevated extracellular levels of myoinositol could impair their breakdown. Either one of these mechanisms could impair phosphoinositide turnover, which may be the key factor in determining the cellular function of this particular pathway.

Dr. Williamson

I was surprised to hear you say you were sad to see that this problem in myoinositol metabolism was not genetic. I would think you might rejoice that it was a complication of the metabolic perturbations which were amenable to treatment.

Dr. Clements

I was being facetious; somewhat analogous to the original discovery of hemoglobin A_{Ic} which initially was thought to be of little importance because it was not a genetic marker for the diabetic state. Nonetheless, both the hemoglobin A_{Ic} and inositol story may prove to be of value in our attempts to elucidate the pathogenesis of diabetic complications.

Dr. Davis

It occurs to me that Dr. James Nelson at Washington University has found that animals maintained on streptozotocin also develop a megacolon with a compromised motility. Now, this may say something about peripheral nerve degenerative changes in diabetic animals. But is it also being accounted for and taken into consideration in, say, the absorptive capacity of various dietary constituents that are being fed the animals that are maintained on streptozotocin?

Dr. Clements

The data on the streptozotocin rats is not quite as complete as on the alloxan diabetic rats who, as I recall, will develop edema of the large bowel if they are maintained for long periods of time. Dr. Daughaday studied the absorption of myoinositol from the gut of normal and diabetic animals using the Cori technique and observed that over a 24-hour period the total absorption of myoinositol is similar in both the diabetic and the nondiabetic rat. So, although your point is quite valid, I don't think there is that much evidence to suggest that there is decreased absorption of myoinositol in the diabetic.

Dr. Werner

Dr. Jackson, would you like to comment on your experience with hemoglobin A_{Ic}?

Dr. Jackson

During the past year, using the method of Trivelli, we have determined A_{Ic} hemoglobin levels in normal subjects, a few diabetics in "poor" control, a number of children with recent onset of overt diabetes, and selected children with diabetes maintained in higher degrees of control. A_{Ic} hemoglobin values for our normal subjects were well within the lower range of 3% to 6% reported in the literature by other research laboratories. All diabetic subjects in "poor" control and children with recent onset, prior to treatment, had elevated values of over 10%. The A_{Ic} values of all children with recent onset of diabetes, maintained in optimum metabolic control, decreased gradually to within the normal range in about eight weeks. In our experience, it is easy to identify and classify with confidence children with diabetes who maintain higher degrees of diabetic control. The children in "good" control selected for study had reliable home records, were essentially aglycosuric and had normal, or only slightly elevated, blood sugar values at clinic visits three to five times per year. A_{Ic} hemoglobin values of these children with diabetes, five to 18 years of age, maintained in "good" control for a few months, and some of them for many years, were less than 6%. Patients with more recent onset requiring less than 0.3 units of insulin/*kg/day* had lower values than the patients with longer duration requiring 0.3 to 0.9 units of insulin/*kg/day*.

It is generally believed and stated in the literature that it is impossible to attain and maintain a sufficient degree of control of diabetes in children to revert and sustain the A_{Ic} hemoglobin level within the normal range. From the above observations, we know that this is not so. However, I would like to stress that most of the children with overt insulin-dependent diabetes with normal A_{Ic} hemoglobin levels are those patients who have been maintained in partial remission by early diagnosis, intensive education of the family, and physiological management in order to control glycosuria.

Dr. Werner

One of the problems that has been mentioned with the hemoglobin A_{Ic} is the very small differences between normals and some of the diabetic patients. I am wondering if either you or Dr. Peterson would comment on that particular aspect and whether there are new techniques on the horizon for these same measurements.

Dr. Jackson

We did not discuss that.

Dr. Peterson

I can certainly confirm Dr. Jackson's experience. In New York there are a large number of diabetic patients that are way out of control. In terms of trying to bring juvenile-type diabetics under control, we're trying to do that now with adolescents and young adults who have had diabetes for a long time and who have been out of control for a long time. In our experience, although we are not measuring serum C-peptide, certainly those children or young adults who have insulin requirements of less than 0.7 *units/kg*, that is those whom we would consider in remission, are much easier to maintain in control than those who are requiring higher insulin dosage.

In terms of methodology, there are three classes of methods coming up. One uses columns. We still use the old regular column method of Trivelli (1971). Others have tried to do high pressure liquid chromatography or speed them up in some way (Cole, Bunn, and Soeldner, 1977).

We've also been looking at the method of Fluckiger and Winterhalter (1976) which is a colorimetric assay which quantitates furfural production. It utilizes the old Browning reaction from the dairy industry to look at glycosylation reactions. We have also developed a radioimmunoassay method (Javid, Pettis, Koenig, and Cerami, 1978). I think that by next year there will be a couple of relatively quiet and useful assays for this glycoprotein.

Dr. Werner

Are there other glycosylated intermediates that people are looking at for use in monitoring control?

Dr. Peterson

Well, hemoglobin AI_a and AI_b are both related to diabetes and are probably glycosylated hemoglobins, although their structures have not been defined (Koenig, Peterson, Jones, Saudik, Lehrman, and Cerami, 1976).

DICUSSION REFERENCES

Cerami, A., Koenig, R.J., Peterson, C.M., and Stevens, V.M. 1978. Formation of Hb AI_c as a biochemical model for the sequelae of diabetes. IN George Brewer (Ed.) *Proc. 4th Internat'l. Conf. on Red Cell Metabol. and Funct.*, Ann Arbor, MI. New York: Alan R. Liss, Inc. In press.

Cole, R.A., Bunn, H.F., and Soeldner, J.S. 1977. New rapid assay method for hemoglobin Hb AI_c and total fast (abstract). *Diabetes* 26(Suppl. 1):392.

Fluckiger, R. and Winterhalter, K.H. 1976. *In-vitro* synthesis of hemoglobin AI_c. *FEBS Lett.* 71:356-360.

Javid, J. Pettis, P.K., Koenig, R.J., and Cerami, A. 1978. Immunologic characterization and quantification of Hb AI_c. *Brit. J. Haematol.* **38**:329-337.

Koenig, R.J., Peterson, C.M., Jones, R.L., Saudek, C., Lehrman, M., and Cerami, A. 1976. The correlation of glucose regulation and hemoglobin AI_c in diabetes mellitus. *New Eng. J. Med.* **295**:417-420.

Schmidt, G.E., Martin, A.P., Townsend, J.R., and Vorbeck, M.L. 1977. Basement membrane synthesis in spontaneously diabetic *Mystromys albicaudatus*. *J. Cell Biol.* **75**:155a. (Abstr.)

Stevens, V.S., Vlassara, H., Abati, A., and Cerami, A. 1977. Nonenzymatic glycosylation of hemoglobin. *J. Biol. Chem.* **252**: 2998-3002.

Trivelli, L.A., Ranney, H.M., and Lai, H-T. 1971. Hemoglobin components in patients with diabetes mellitus. *New Eng. J. Med.* **284**:353-357.

BASEMENT MEMBRANES IN MUSCLE CAPILLARIES

C. Kilo and J.R. Williamson

Departments of Pathology and Medicine
Washington University School of Medicine
St. Louis, MO 63110

SUMMARY

Thickening of capillary basement membranes, including those of skeletal muscle, is now widely accepted as the ultrastructural hallmark of diabetic microangiopathy. Although muscle capillary basement membrane thickening has been reported in a limited number of collagen diseases, diabetes mellitus is by far the commonest disease associated with capillary basement membrane thickening. Muscle capillary basement membrane width increases in nondiabetic males essentially throughout life. In nondiabetic females, capillary basement membrane thickening tends to increase less rapidly until after the menopause. In both sexes basement membrane width increases linearly with increasing hydrostatic pressure in muscles below the heart level.

In a series of 138 juvenile-onset diabetics (age 10-24) recently examined, muscle capillary basement membrane width increased significantly with increasing age and with postpubertal duration, but not prepubertal or total duration, of diabetes. These observations indicate that: (1) some, as yet unidentified, puberty-related factor exerts an important permissive effect on muscle capillary basement membrane thickening in diabetic subjects and that (2) muscle capillary basement membrane thickening is, in some way, a consequence of the abnormal metabolic milieu and hormonal imbalances associated with the diabetic state. These interpretations and conclusions are supported by recent studies on monozygotic twins and triplets, discordant for diabetes, which document muscle capillary basement membrane thickening only in those individuals with diabetes.

INTRODUCTION

Cross-sectional studies by numerous investigators are in general agreement that capillary basement membranes of diabetics are thickened in many tissues, including skin, kidney, and skeletal muscle (see review by Williamson and Kilo, 1977), and thickening of capillary basement membrane is widely accepted as the ultrastructural hallmark of diabetic microangiopathy. On the other hand, the prevalence of capillary basement membrane thickening in diabetics and its pathogenetic relationships to the metabolic and hormonal imbalances of diabetes have been the subject of considerable controversy.

In this report we will discuss, very briefly, some of the structural and functional properties of muscle capillary basement membrane in nondiabetics as well as in diabetics and we will consider some of the proposed mechanisms of pathogenesis and the pathophysiological consequences of capillary basement membrane thickening in diabetics.

Muscle Capillary Basement Membranes in Nondiabetics

Very significant age-related changes in capillary basement membrane occur in nondiabetic subjects. These changes may have important implications regarding the pathogenesis of capillary basement membrane thickening in diabetics. At birth, capillary basement membranes of pectoral, abdominal wall, thigh, and calf muscles are of comparable width (Williamson, Vogler, and Kilo, 1971) and increase in width in all these muscles with age. However, by age 3 or 4, capillary basement membranes of muscles in the lower extremity are appreciably thicker than those of pectoral and abdominal wall, and by adulthood, capillary basement membranes of calf muscle are approximately two times thicker than those of abdominal wall muscle. It is of interest that capillary basement membrane width of muscles below heart level increases linearly with increasing venous hydrostatic pressure. This suggests that capillary basement membrane thickening may, in some way, be mediated by an increase in vascular pressure and/or by physiological changes in functional properties of vessels associated with increased vascular pressure.

It is also of interest that significant age-related sex differences are demonstrable in capillary basement membrane width of nondiabetic subjects (Kilo, Vogler, and Williamson, 1972). During the period of approximately 30-50 years of age, capillary basement membrane width in males is significantly thicker than in females. However, after the menopause capillary basement membranes thicken rapidly in females to catch up with those of males. These observations suggest that sex-hormone-related factors exert a significant influence on muscle capillary basement membrane thickening.

A characteristic feature of capillary basement membrane thickening in nondiabetics, which is also true for diabetics, is that the thickening is quite uneven. It tends to vary in width around the circumference as well as along the length of the vessel (Kilo *et al.*, 1972). Thus, when viewed in cross-section, some vessels manifest thickened basement membrane around the entire circumference whereas others have basement membrane of normal width around the entire circumference.

Muscle Capillary Basement Membranes in Diabetics

Although cross-sectional studies of muscle capillary basement membranes in diabetics have, in general, confirmed that basement membranes are much thicker than in nondiabetics, both the magnitude of basement membrane thickening and the frequency with which thickened basement membranes are observed have varied considerably in different series (reviewed in Williamson and Kilo, 1977). Although some investigators have attributed this variability in results to differences in fixatives and differences in morphometric techniques employed to assess capillary basement membrane width (Siperstein, Raskin, and Burns, 1973), the observations cited in support of this explanation are subject to serious criticisms and have not been substantiated by other investigators (Williamson and Kilo, 1977; Williamson, Rowold, Hoffman, and Kilo, 1976a). A more likely explanation, in our opinion, is the fact that most of these studies were performed on maturity onset diabetics in whom it is well recognized that the time of onset of insulin deficiency and carbohydrate intolerance cannot be accurately dated. Thus, many of these diabetics may have "asymptomatic" mild to moderate carbohydrate intolerance for many years prior to the time diabetes is diagnosed. This would also account for the finding that capillary basement membrane thickening may be present at the time diabetes is diagnosed in these subjects.

Studies of the frequency of muscle capillary basement membrane thickening and its relationship to duration of diabetes are much more meaningful when conducted on subjects in whom the onset of diabetes can be dated with some accuracy, as in juvenile-onset diabetics in whom the margin of error in dating the onset of diabetes is reduced by virtue of: (1) the younger age of the group under study and (2) the onset of the diabetic state which is generally acknowledged to be much more abrupt in this type of diabetes than in adults.

All except one group of investigators have reported that the frequency of capillary basement membrane thickening in newly diagnosed juvenile-onset diabetics is quite low (approximately 10%).

Observations from our laboratory indicate that the frequency and magnitude of muscle capillary basement membrane thickening in juvenile-onset diabetics between ages 10-25 increases with age and with postpubertal, but not prepubertal, duration of diabetes. In contrast, capillary basement membrane thickness does not increase with age in control subjects in this age range matched for age and sex. These observations suggest that some puberty-related factor exerts an important permissive effect on the development of muscle capillary basement membrane thickening in diabetes.

Important questions regarding: (1) the influence of the severity of the diabetic state, *i.e.*, mean 24-hour blood glucose level and (2) whether capillary basement membrane thickening is reversible, are still not adequately answered. Recent observations reported by two groups of investigators (Jackson, Gutherie, Esterly, Bilginturan, James, Yeast, Saathoff, and Guthrie, 1975; Sheikholislam, Irias, Lin, Lowrey, Stephenson, Peterson, Devereux, and Volk, 1976; Sheikholislam, Irias, Lowrey, and Lin, 1976) suggest that muscle capillary basement membrane thickening in diabetic state and that it is reversible. Both of these studies are based on small numbers of subjects and must be substantiated in larger series.

PATHOGENESIS AND PATHOPHYSIOLOGICAL SIGNIFICANCE OF MUSCLE CAPILLARY BASEMENT MEMBRANE THICKENING

The observations just discussed are consistent with the hypothesis that muscle capillary basement membrane thickening in diabetes is somehow a consequence of the abnormal metabolic milieu and hormonal imbalances which characterize the diabetic state. On the other hand, some investigators have suggested that genetic factors independent of those responsible for the abnormal metabolic milieu and hormonal imbalances might govern capillary basement membrane thickening and diabetic vascular disease in general. If this were true, it has been postulated that such genes for vascular disease might be manifested occasionally in the absence of diabetes in individuals with a strong hereditary background for diabetes, *i.e.*, in the nondiabetic offspring of two diabetic parents and in the nondiabetic member of identical twins discordant for diabetes. In general, it can be said that the prevalence of capillary basement membrane thickening in cross-sectional studies of nondiabetic offspring of diabetic parents is low and that even those individuals who do manifest capillary basement membrane thickening may have had carbohydrate intolerance in the past (Williamson and Kilo, 1977). It is of considerable interest that of the published reports on a single set of identical twins (Karam, Rosenthal, O'Donnell, Tsalikian, Lorenzi, Gerich, Siperstein, and Forsham, 1977) and a single set of monozygotic triplets discordant for diabetes

(Ganda, Soeldner, Gleason, Smith, Kilo, and Williamson, 1977), only the diabetic members have manifested evidence of muscle capillary basement membrane thickening. Thus, at the present time, there is essentially no evidence to support the existence of genetic determinants for vascular disease specific to diabetes. It is important to emphasize, however, that there may well be genetically-determined factors present in the general population which, when superimposed on the diabetic state, may influence the pathogenesis, the progression, and the severity of diabetic vascular disease (Pyke and Tattersall, 1973).

The molecular and cellular mechanisms involved in mediating the effects of the diabetic milieu on blood vessels and vascular disease remain to be identified. The fact that several factors can influence muscle capillary basement membrane width in nondiabetics suggests that the pathogenesis of diabetic vascular disease may be multifactorial. The interrelationships between vascular pressure, vascular permeability, and capillary basement membrane thickening are especially intriguing (reviewed in Williamson and Kilo, 1976b, 1977).

Observations in nondiabetics indicate that vascular permeability is increased in subjects with increased vascular pressure. In fact, most of the risk factors for large vessel disease are associated with increased vascular permeability. Thus, it is reasonable to suggest that the increase in capillary basement membrane width in the lower extremity of nondiabetic subjects may be a consequence of increased vascular permeability associated with increased vascular pressure.

If increased vascular permeability is a causative factor in capillary basement membrane thickening in the lower extremity of nondiabetics, this same mechanism could account for generalized capillary basement membrane thickening in diabetics in whom increased vascular permeability is well documented (Williamson and Kilo, 1977). On the other hand, an explanation is still needed for the increased vascular permeability in diabetes. It is important to note that if capillary basement membrane thickening in diabetics is mediated by acceleration of the same cellular mechanisms responsible for capillary basement membrane thickening in the lower extremity of nondiabetics, then it is not surprising that no more than subtle changes have been reported in the composition of glomerular basement membrane isolated from diabetic subjects (see review by Williamson and Kilo, 1977). It is also evident that since muscle capillary basement membrane thickening in the lower extremity of nondiabetics occurs in the absence of the diabetic milieu, basement membrane thickening in the diabetic need not be a direct consequence of the abnormal metabolic milieu on basement membrane synthesis or degradation.

Increased vascular permeability could conceivably lead to excess basement membrane accumulation by two mechanisms. First, leakage of plasma inhibitors of collagenase, such as alpha-1-antitrypsin and alpha-2-macroglobulin could interfere with degradation of basement membrane which is a member of the collagen family of proteins. Second, activation of plasma factors leaked into the perivascular space could stimulate increased synthesis of capillary basement membrane in a manner analogous to stimulation of collagen production at sites of injury and wound healing where vascular permeability is also markedly increased.

Thickened muscle capillary basement membranes in diabetics have been postulated to (1) be more permeable than normal, thus accounting for proteinuria; (2) interfere with movement of hormones, *i.e.*, insulin, and exchange of nutrients across vessel walls; and (3) interfere with migration of leukocytes through vessel walls and contribute to increased susceptibility of diabetics to infections.

In regard to the first postulate we would point out that in most tissues, endothelium rather than capillary basement membrane, is rate limiting to the molecular markers for which permeability has been shown to be increased in diabetics. Therefore, we would suggest that the evidence available is more consistent with the concept that increased vascular permeability in diabetics is due to compromised integrity of endothelial cells rather than of basement membrane. Because of the unique structure and functional properties of the glomerulus, the relative importance of epithelial foot processes, basement membrane, and endothelium as determinants of glomerular permeability remains somewhat controversial.

For the reasons just cited, plus the documented increase in vascular permeability, the second postulate that diffusion of hormones and metabolites etc. may be hindered in diabetics is untenable. Although there is no direct evidence in support of the third postulate, it seems very likely that capillary basement membrane thickening could, indeed, interfere with migration of leukocytes through vessel walls.

ACKNOWLEDGMENT

We would like to acknowledge the support of the Charles Kilo Diabetes and Vascular Diseases Research Foundation and USPHS grant 13694.

REFERENCES

Ganda, O.M., Soeldner, J.S., Gleason, R.E., Smith, T.M., Kilo, C., and Williamson, J.R. 1977. Monozygotic triplets with discordance for diabetes mellitus and diabetic microangiopathy. *Diabetes* 26:469-479.

Jackson, R., Guthrie, R., Esterly, J., Bilginturan, N., James, R., Yeast, J., Saathoff, J., and Guthrie, D. 1975. Muscle capillary basement membrane changes in normal and diabetic children. *Diabetes* 24(Suppl. 2):400 (Abstr.).

Karam, J.H., Rosenthal, M., O'Donnell, J.J., Tsalikian, E., Lorenzi, M., Gerich, J.E., Siperstein, M.D., and Forsham, P.H. 1977. Discordance of diabetic microangiopathy in identical twins. *Diabetes* 25:24-28.

Kilo, C., Vogler, N., and Williamson, J.R. 1972. Muscle capillary basement membrane changes related to aging and to diabetes mellitus. *Diabetes* 21:881-905.

Pyke, D.A. and Tattersall, R.B. 1973. Diabetic retinopathy in identical twins. *Diabetes* 22:613-618.

Sheikholislam, B.M., Irias, J.J., Lin, H-J, Lowrey, G.H., Stephenson, S.R., Peterson, G.E., Devereux, D.F., and Volk, T.L. 1976. Carbohydrate metabolism and capillary basement-membrane thickness in children. I. Cross-sectional studies. *Diabetes* 25:650-660.

Sheikholislam, B.M., Irias, J.J., Lowrey, G.H., and Lin, H-J. 1976. Carbohydrate metabolism and capillary basement-membrane thickness in children. II. Longitudinal studies. *Diabetes* 25:661-666.

Siperstein, M.D., Raskin, P., and Burns, H. 1973. Electron microscopic quantification of diabetic microangiopathy. *Diabetes* 22:514-527.

Williamson, J.R. and Kilo, C. 1976. Basement-membrane thickening and diabetic microangiopathy. *Diabetes* 25(Suppl. 2):925-927.

Williamson, J.R. and Kilo, C. 1977. Current status of capillary basement-membrane disease in diabetes mellitus. *Diabetes* 26: 65-75.

Williamson, J.R., Rowold, E., Hoffman, P., and Kilo, C. 1976. Influence of fixation and morphometric technics on capillary basement-membrane thickening prevalence data in diabetes. *Diabetes* 25:604-613.

Williamson, J.R., Vogler, N.J., and Kilo, C. 1971. Regional variations in the width of the basement membrane of muscle capillaries in man and giraffe. *Am. J. Path.* 63:359-367.

BIOCHEMISTRY OF THE BASEMENT MEMBRANE IN DIABETES MELLITUS

Michael Brownlee and Robert G. Spiro

Harvard Medical School
Elliot P. Joslin Research Laboratory
170 Pilgrim Road
Boston, MA 02215

OUTLINE

Introduction

Chemical Characterization of Glomerular Basement Membrane

Changes in Diabetes Mellitus

Variations in Methodology

Variations in Clinical-Pathological Characteristics of Diabetic Kidneys Studied

Biosynthesis and Degradation of Glomerular Basement Membrane

Glycosyltransferases

Amino-Acid Incorporation

Pathophysiology of Basement Membrane Changes in Diabetes Mellitus

Conclusions

INTRODUCTION

In recent years, extensive investigations have demonstrated that numerous biochemical and physiological abnormalities occur in various tissues of hyperglycemic animals and humans (Brownlee and Cahill, 1979). Where the effect of treatment has been studied, many, if not all of these abnormalities, are returned towards normal with insulin, and it seems likely that some of these may play a role in the pathogenesis of diabetic renal disease. Others are likely to be mere concomitants of the microvascular disease which reflect common metabolic abnormalities of the diabetic state, but are causally unrelated. Although it appears increasingly likely that the morphological and clinical features of diabetic nephropathy result from a complex combination of interacting variables, the relative significance of individual factors is currently unknown. Whatever the sequence of events leading from abnormal glucose homeostasis to progressive renal failure with persistent proteinuria, the final clinical manifestations reflect irreversible glomerular capillary occlusion and increased permeability of the glomerular filtration barrier. Both of these result from alterations in basement membrane. The accumulation of basement membrane material having altered filtration properties, thus, represents the ultimate structural and functional basis of diabetic renal disease.

Although much information about the biochemistry of the glomerular basement membrane has been obtained (Cohen and Klein, 1979; Spiro, 1976; Taylor and Price, 1977; Westberg and Michael, 1970), discordant reports concerning the effects of diabetes on this structure have caused an understandable degree of confusion among diabetologists (Beisswenger, 1976; Beisswenger and Spiro, 1970;Cohen and Khalifa, 1977; Cohen and Vogt, 1975b; Grant, Harwood, and Williams, 1976; Kefalides, 1974; Khalifa and Cohen, 1975; Risteli, Koivisto, and Akerblom, 1976; Spiro, 1976; Spiro and Spiro, 1971a). Because a correct understanding of the structure and metabolism of glomerular basement membrane is an essential prerequisite to any further elucidation of the process of diabetic glomerular disease, this discussion will focus critically on the experimental basis for these reported discrepancies, in the course of reviewing and summarizing current knowledge of basement membrane biochemistry.

CHEMICAL CHARACTERIZATION OF GLOMERULAR BASEMENT MEMBRANE

Over the past decade, much information about the chemical structure of the normal glomerular basement membrane has been acquired. Although much of the basic structural work was done on bovine material, compositional studies performed in several mammalian species have yielded similar results (Beisswenger and Spiro, 1973; Price and Spiro, 1977; Sato and Spiro, 1976). The basement membrane is composed of collagen-like glycoprotein material, being particularly rich in the amino acids glycine, hydroxyproline, and hydroxylysine. However, it clearly differs from fibrillar collagen, since it contains three times as much hydroxylysine, large amounts of half-cystine, and has a significant carbohydrate content (Spiro, 1976). Recent analysis of the Clq component of complement has shown a very similar composition for this soluble serum protein (Reid, 1974). The sugar constituents of the basement membrane are distributed between two distinct types of carbohydrate units (Spiro, 1967b). One is a complex asparagine-linked heteropolysaccharide containing galactose, mannose, fucose, sialic acid, and glucosamine, occurring on relatively more polar, less collagen-like portions of the peptide chain. These heteropolysaccharide units are not particularly characteristic of basement membrane, and have been described in a variety of other glycoproteins (Spiro, 1973a).

The second type of carbohydrate unit consists of a glucose-galactose disaccharide unit attached to hydroxylysine. The two carbohydrate units are found in a ratio of 1:10 by number, but by total weight are about equal. Hydroxylysine is formed by the enzymatic hydroxylation of lysine residues that are already incorporated in nascent or released polypeptides. Eighty percent of this hydroxylysine is then linked to galactose and, subsequently, to glucose by sequential sugar transferase enzymes to form the disaccharide-hydroxylysine complex (Spiro, 1973b).

After reduction of its disulfide cross-links, the basement membrane can be solubilized in SDS or urea and, subsequently, fractionated into a large number of components spanning the molecular weight range from 25,000 to over 200,000 *daltons* (Hudson and Spiro, 1972a, 1972b; Sato and Spiro, 1976). These subunits vary greatly in their amino acid and carbohydrate composition. Some are rich in the collagen-like components, while others contain more polar amino acids such as half-cystine, tyrosine, and aspartic acid. Most subunits contain both types of carbohydrate units, but in quite different proportions. Even material of the same molecular size exhibits this compositional heterogeneity. Although the basis for this subunit polydispersity is unknown, it has been shown that these various polypeptides do not arise by proteolytic cleavage of a high molecular weight component during membrane isolation (Cohen and Klein, 1976; Freytag, Ohno, and Hudson, 1976). Rather, they may be the result of a limited physiologic *in vivo* proteolytic digestion of a smaller number of large basement membrane subunits (Spiro, 1976).

CHANGES IN DIABETES MELLITUS

Chemical composition studies of human glomerular basement membrane in normal and diabetic kidneys have been published by several groups of investigators (Beisswenger and Spiro, 1970; Kefalides, 1974; Westberg and Michael, 1973). Studies from this laboratory first demonstrated an increased amount of basement membrane-like material in glomeruli from long-term diabetics with microscopically evident nephropathy. In addition, it was found that this material had a distinctly different composition from normal (Beisswenger, 1973; Beisswenger and Spiro, 1973). Compared to the normal, there was increased hydroxylysine with a proportional decrease in lysine, so that the sum of the two remained constant. Glucose and galactose were likewise elevated in the diabetic membrane, corresponding to an increase in hydroxylysine-linked disaccharide residues. Smaller, but still significant, increases of hydroxyproline and glycine were also found, as were decreases in valine and tyrosine. These compositional data suggest that there is an increased presence of hydroxylysine-rich subunits with collagen-like amino acid composition in the diabetic basement membrane. These studies have, subsequently, been confirmed by DeOlivera and Canivet (1976).

In two other studies (Kefalides, 1974; Westberg and Michael, 1973), these differences were not observed. However, a significant decrease in the half-cystine and sialic acid content of glomerular basement membrane (GBM) from diabetic kidneys was noted. Important differences, both in technique of basement membrane preparation and in the diabetic kidneys selected for study, may explain these apparent discrepancies.

VARIATIONS IN METHODOLOGY

A brief consideration of the methodology will provide a useful background for critically interpreting these reported analytical data.

Glomeruli are isolated and purified from kidney cortex by a series of sieving steps through different mesh sizes. Tissue disruption is accomplished by pushing cortex slices through a coarse sieve. Subsequently, selective filtration through coupled sieves results in a separation of glomeruli from other cortical elements. Final centrifugation after generous washing yields a pure glomerular pellet overlaid with Bowman's capsular material (Spiro, 1967a). Omitting any of these sieve passages results in a less complete separation of fibrillar elements and tubules from the isolated glomeruli. Since the unmodified Krakower-Greenspon isolation procedure used by some (Kefalides, 1974) employs only the initial tissue-disruption sieving step, contamination of such glomerular preparations is likely. Since fibrillar collagen is relatively low in hydroxylysine and glucose, any of this material mixing with the basement membrane prepared from such glomeruli would tend to decrease hydroxylysine and glucose content.

Selection of the mesh size of the sieves may also be extremely important, since recent glomerular fractionation experiments (Butcher, Kikkawa, Klein, and Miller, 1977) have demonstrated that glomeruli isolated from human diabetics are distributed among four major groups according to size, while normal glomeruli are equally distributed between two groups. Electron microscopic analysis of glomerular size and structure in long-term diabetes has shown hypertrophied, enlarged glomeruli with nonoccluded capillaries coexisting with another subpopulation of severely diseased glomeruli with capillary occlusion (Gunderson and Osterby, 1977). Thus, improper choice of pore size could exclude the most severely involved glomeruli from analysis.

Basement membrane is isolated and purified from glomeruli by ultrasonication. This mechanical disruption effectively removes cellular contamination from the basement membrane, as assessed by low levels of cellular markers such as DNA, RNA, and most importantly, phospholipid phosphorus (Spiro, 1967a). Since the phospholipid phosphorus derives primarily from the plasma membrane of glomerular cells, it serves as a useful estimate of preparation contamination, inversely correlating with the purity of basement membrane as expressed by the ratio of hydroxylysine to lysine (Westberg and Michael, 1970). It is important, when comparing diabetic and normal basement membrane, to assure equivalent degrees of purity in the two preparations. Otherwise, compositional alterations due to plasma membrane constituents such as sialic acid may erroneously be attributed to changes in the basement membrane itself.

Once cellular contaminants are removed, additional ultrasonication of the basement membrane does not result in any compositional change (Spiro, 1976). In studies reporting increased concentrations of hydroxylysine, hydroxyproline, and glycine after additional sonication (Kefalides, 1974), it seems likely that the original basement membrane preparation represents incompletely disrupted and, therefore, contaminated material.

Significant differences in glomerular basement membrane composition from diabetic kidneys may also result from a modification of the ultrasonication procedure adopted by some groups, in which hyalinized and undisrupted glomeruli are removed from the sonication preparation by an additional sieving step (Westberg and Michael, 1973). Since the average number of hyalinized glomeruli in biopsy material from affected diabetic kidneys is greater than 50% in some series, exclusion of this component may significantly affect the analysis. Indeed, groups employing this preparative modification report that a large percentage of glomeruli are thus removed from the material being analyzed.

VARIATIONS IN THE CLINICAL-PATHOLOGICAL CHARACTERISTICS OF DIABETIC KIDNEYS STUDIED

In addition to important technical differences in basement membrane preparation, differences in the clinical and pathological characteristics of the diabetic kidneys selected for study could also account for some reported negative findings. Since basement membrane turnover is very slow, membrane isolated from diabetics includes material which was synthesized both before and after the onset of the metabolic derangement (Price and Spiro, 1977; Spiro, 1976). Thus, changes which may occur in the composition of the diabetic membrane would be minimized in these analyses by the presence of varying amounts of normal basement membrane material. The magnitude of this dilutional effect can be appreciated by considering the calculated amino acid composition of the hypothetical basement membrane in which 25% of the total is contributed by hydroxylysine-rich, collagen-like subunits. Although such a membrane would be expected to differ from normal only in those subunit constituents which differ most strikingly from that of the whole membrane, it has been calculated that even in these components the hypothetical membrane would show only modest changes from normal (Spiro, 1976). A comparison of the ratios of this hypothetical basement membrane to normal with the ratios of experimentally observed diabetic to normal shows marked similarities for many of the amino acids. Thus, a very substantial subunit derangement in the basement membrane could well result in only a slight alteration of the whole membrane composition. Because total compositional studies of glomerular basement membrane are a rather insensitive index of disease-induced synthetic changes, it is imperative that glomeruli with confirmed pathological alterations be included in the analyses of diabetic tissue. Analyses of diabetic kidney material without microscopic evidence of glomerular disease have not demonstrated chemical abnormalities (Beisswenger, 1973). In addition to using kidney material with diabetic glomerular changes present histologically, it may also be important to compare diabetic and normal individuals who are age-matched. Extrapolating from rat data (Hoyer and Spiro, 1978), it would appear that the glomerular basement membrane hydroxylysine/lysine ratio increases with age. Failure to take this into account may obscure some real compositional differences between normal and diabetic samples.

In the sucrose-fed rat model of diabetic nephropathy, all of these technical factors have been taken into consideration. Recent chemical analysis of these glomerular basement membranes has shown increased hydroxylysine-linked dissacharide units quite similar to the findings in human diabetic glomerular basement membrane (Price, personal communication).

BIOSYNTHESIS AND DEGRADATION OF GLOMERULAR BASEMENT MEMBRANE

The compositional abnormalities discussed in the previous section may be partially responsible for the altered filtration properties of the glomerular basement membrane in diabetes which, ultimately, result in clinically significant continuous, nonselective proteinuria. It is speculated that increased glycosylation might interfere with polypeptide packing and/or lysine-derived cross-link formation, due to steric hindrance by the bulky carbohydrate groups. This might result in an increased effective pore size of the basement membrane. Other, more subtle, compositional changes undetectable by total membrane analysis could also be significant in this regard.

While the proteinuric component of diabetic nephropathy no doubt reflects changes in the structure of the basement membrane, the progressive fall in glomerular filtration rate (GFR) with chronic renal failure is a consequence of the abnormal accumulation of excessive amounts of basement membrane material with resultant glomerular capillary occlusion. This excessive accumulation of GBM in diabetes could represent increased synthesis, decreased degradation, or a combination of the two processes. Increases in basement membrane synthesis could affect all subunits equally. Alternatively, there could be a relative overproduction of selected basement membrane components. Similarly, degradation may be uniform and nonspecific, or it may affect some portions of the basement membrane preferentially. Such differential subunit effects, if they do occur, could account for the qualitative, as well as quantitative alterations in diabetic glomerular basement membrane. Compositional analysis, however, would be a relatively insensitive means of detecting these changes.

Metabolic studies of GBM have, by necessity, been limited to animal systems. Although the appropriateness of the rat model has been questioned by some investigators (Klein, Yoshida, and Miller, 1977), recent work has established that experimental diabetes results in increased kidney protein content and protein/DNA ratio, as well as significant glomerular capillary basement membrane thickening (Fox and Darby, 1977; Osterby, 1978; Seyer-Hansen, 1977; Yagihashi, Goto, Kakizaki, and Kaseda, 1978). A highly significant, positive correlation exists between these parameters and the degree of hyperglycemia. Low carbohydrate diet plus insulin administration reduce the basement membrane thickening (Fox and Darby, 1977).

Kidney ribosome preparations from rats made diabetic with alloxan, streptozotocin, or anti-insulin serum incorporate amino acids into protein at a greater rate than do ribosomes prepared from normal rat kidney (Peterson, Greene, and Reaven, 1971). This observation suggests that diabetes leads to increased kidney protein synthesis.

GLYCOSYLTRANSFERASES

Indirect evidence for accelerated glomerular basement membrane biosynthesis in diabetic kidney comes from studies of enzymes involved in the assembly of its hydroxylysine-linked disaccharide units. These units are synthesized by a series of specific enzymatic, postribosomal steps. The first involves the hydroxylation of lysine residues that are already incorporated in the newly synthesized peptide chains (Spiro, 1973b). Evidence has been presented which suggests that lysyl hydroxylase activity is increased in the soluble fraction of kidney homogenates from diabetic animals (Khalifa and Cohen, 1975). However, this enzyme has not yet been isolated and characterized adequately enough to permit definite conclusions.

After the hydroxylation of lysine, the sequential participation of two very specific glycosyltransferases completes the synthetic process. One is a galactosyltransferase which functions only to transfer galactose from the activated sugar UDP-galactose to hydroxylysine in high molecular weight components (Spiro and Spiro, 1971c). The other is a glucosyltransferase which only transfers glucose to hydroxylysine-linked galactose (Spiro and Spiro, 1971b). In contrast to the hydroxylase, both of these enzymes have been intensively investigated and extremely well characterized in the rat renal cortex, using "glucose-free" and "disaccharide-free" GBM as the enzyme substrates. Purified hydroxylysine-linked disaccharide units synthesized in the assay system were isolated by ion-exchange and paper chromatography prior to determination of enzymatic specific activities. The activity of the specific basement membrane glucosyltransferase varies markedly with age, reaching a peak at nine days and then falling rapidly to lower levels as the animal matures (Spiro and Spiro, 1971b). In kidney cortex from diabetic rats, the activity of this enzyme is significantly elevated over that of age-matched normal controls, and this difference increases with the duration of the disease. Simultaneous measurements of glucosyltransferase activity in several other tissues of the diabetic rats do not show any differences from normal (Spiro and Spiro, 1971a). Moreover, measurement of another kidney glycosyltransferase enzyme, one involved in the synthesis of the heteropolysaccharide unit of the basement membrane, also shows no difference from normal. The observed elevation of renal glucosyltransferase activity in the diabetic animals most likely reflects a specific increase in GBM synthetic activity.

This finding has been challenged by Risteli, Koivisto, and Akerblom (1976), who reported no changes in glycosyltransferase activity after either four weeks or 12 weeks of streptozotocin diabetes. When their results are expressed as total enzyme activity per kidney, rather than activity per *milligram* of protein, however, significant increases are observed after 12 weeks of diabetes.

The assay system developed by Spiro utilizes glomerular basement membrane-glycopeptides with selected sugars removed as acceptors for the GBM glycosyltransferases. In contrast, Risteli *et al.* employ the less specific gelatinized collagen. This methodological difference could significantly reduce the specificity of the Koivisto enzyme assay and, thus, diminish the ability to discriminate between basement membrane glycosyltransferases and other renal (*e.g.*, collagen) sugar transferases. Using glomerular basement membrane glycopeptides as substrate, Price (personal communication) and others recently demonstrated increased disaccharide-synthesizing glycosyltransferases in the kidney cortex of sucrose-fed rats, an animal model of diabetic glomerular disease.

AMINO-ACID INCORPORATION

While studies of glycosyltransferase activities provide indirect evidence suggesting accelerated glomerular basement membrane synthesis in diabetes, more direct evidence comes from investigations of amino acid incorporation into glomerular proteins. Incubations of isolated rat golmeruli have been utilized in several studies of basement membrane biosynthesis, both in normal and in diabetic animals (Beisswenger, 1976; Cohen and Vogt, 1972, 1975a; Grant, Harwood, and Williams, 1975, 1976). Great caution must be exercised in the interpretation of such studies, however, because of serious problems with the metabolic properties of these preparations. Although these glomeruli are viable as determined with trypan blue, there is a serious but apparently overlooked difficulty with the normal basement membrane synthetic process in such systems (Price and Spiro, 1977). Basement membrane hydroxylysine and hydroxyproline result from enzymatic hydroxylation of lysine and proline, respectively, after it is incorporated into the nascent peptide chain. Therefore, the ratio of the specific activity of hydroxylysine to lysine, and of hydroxyproline to proline, should approximate unity. While this information is lacking in most published reports, a useful estimation can be made from the ratios of hydroxylysine *cpm* to lysine plus hydroxylysine *cpm* (or similarly for hydroxyproline and proline) which one can calculate from the available data. Since rat renal basement membrane contains 20.6 residues of hydroxylysine, 23.8 residues of lysine, 69.5 residues of hydroxyproline, and 73.5 residues of proline per 1,000 amino acid residues, these calculated ratios should approach .46 and .49. In the work of Grant *et al.* (1975), this ratio for proline varies between .02 and .05. Although these authors have, subsequently, reported an increased synthesis of GBM in streptozotocin diabetes (Grant *et al.*, 1976), the physiological meaning of this is unclear.

Similarly, the calculated values for hydroxylysine and lysine *cpm* reported by Beisswenger (1976) are also in the range of .02. In contrast to Grant *et al.* (1975), recovery of label in hydroxylysine of diabetic GBM did not differ from controls. Beyond the observation that neither preparation is synthesizing and hydroxylating GBM properly, however, no conclusions can be justifiably made. Although Cohen and Vogt (1975a) have obtained a more favorable ratio of .19 hydroxylysine in their glomerular culture system, this is still less than half of the normal value. Therefore, although they also observed an increased basement membrane synthesis in diabetic glomeruli (Cohen and Vogt, 1972), the same caveats mentioned previously apply here as well. Even if isolated glomerular systems did function normally, it could still be argued that interpretation and extrapolation of such data would be difficult, due to the artificial, nonphysiologic incubation milieu. Consequently, intact animal studies have been undertaken in an effort to circumvent these difficulties.

Lazarow and Speidel (1964) attempted to compare proline incorporation into normal and diabetic glomerular basement membrane. They reported that the specific activity of both proline and hydroxyproline was less in the diabetic than in the control animals. In addition, they noted persistence of radioactivity in the diabetic preparation after detectable counts had disappeared from the normals. These observations were interpreted as evidence for decreased synthesis and decreased degradation in diabetic animals. Unfortunately, there is no convincing evidence that the material studied by these investigators was, in fact, glomerular basement membrane. There are no adequate analyses of amino acid composition, nor are there chemical determinations of preparation purity such as phospholipid phosphorus content. In addition, the material studied by Lazarow and Speidel was insoluble in NaOH, while glomerular basement membrane is almost completely solubilized under similar conditions. It, thus, seems extremely unlikely that this study represents incorporation of radioactive precursors into glomerular basement membrane. An additional neglected factor of major importance in any *in vivo* comparative study is the specific activity of the precursor proline pool in the diabetic and control animals. Failure to obtain and correct for this data would render subsequent conclusions invalid.

Recent careful *in vivo* studies of normal glomerular basement membrane turnover have been performed by Price and Spiro, utilizing injected tracer doses of tritiated amino acids. The rat glomerular basement membrane in this study was well characterized by amino acid composition and by chemical assessment of cellular contamination (Price and Spiro, 1977). In these studies, the ratio of proline to hydroxyproline specific activity approached unity, indicating normal synthesis and hydroxylation. Basement membrane turnover rates were determined from the decay in specific activity of a number of incorporated amino acids. Data from the specific activity of glomerular basement membrane proline and hydroxyproline indicate that the turnover rate of GBM is extremely slow in comparison to other glomerular proteins, approaching that of fibrillar collagen. Additional data from the specific activity of other amino acids suggest that GBM polypeptide components of dissimilar composition may turn over at different rates.

Utilizing injected tracer doses of tritiated proline, Brownlee and Spiro (1979) have extended these analyses to include comparative data from diabetic and normal rats. Preliminary investigations revealed a significant difference in the specific activity of the precursor proline pool between the two groups of animals. This finding of substantially decreased proline-specific activity in the serum of diabetic animals may represent dilution by an increased peripheral output of the unlabeled amino acid to meet the demands of augmented gluconeogenesis. A valid comparison of *in vivo* basement membrane synthesis between normal and diabetic animals could not be made without taking into account these differences in the specific activity of the injected radiolabeled amino acid in the precursor pools.

In this *in vivo* animal model, the incorporation of radioactivity into the basement membrane of both normals and diabetics was slow, and a period of almost constant specific activity of proline and hydroxyproline was observed after maximum incorporation was reached. In the diabetic basement membrane, however, the specific activity of both these amino acids was nearly twice that attained in normal basement membrane. These results are consistent with accelerated rates of glomerular basement membrane polypeptide synthesis and proline hydroxylation in diabetes, and constitute the most direct evidence presently available in support of this hypothesis.

PATHOPHYSIOLOGY OF BASEMENT MEMBRANE CHANGES IN DIABETES MELLITUS

A conceptual framework for understanding the alterations in basement membrane synthesis which occur in diabetes is provided by the following considerations. Only certain tissues require insulin for the intracellular transport or phosphorylation of glucose (Spiro, 1971). Other tissues, including kidney, do not, and thus equilibrate with the extracellular glucose concentration. Hyperglycemia would, therefore, produce an elevated glucose concentration within the cells of such tissues. This effect would be magnified in diabetes by both a shunting of glucose from insulin-dependent to insulin-independent tissues, and by an increased glucose release from the liver. The resulting high glucose concentration in glomerular cells could significantly affect basement membrane synthesis in two ways. First, because glycosylation of hydroxylysine in the peptide chain is a postribosomal synthetic step, availability of sugar substrate may well be an important rate-limiting factor in the regulation of basement membrane disaccharide synthesis (Rasio and Bendayan, 1978). In addition to increasing the synthesis of disaccharide units, high glucose concentrations may well have a direct effect on the synthesis and secretion of the peptide portion of basement membrane as well. The data derived from diabetic rats, discussed above, is consistent with this notion. Additional support for this effect of hyperglycemia comes from recent observations of collagen secretion by human skin fibroblasts *in vitro* (Villee and Lowers, 1977). Cells growing in a high glucose medium secreted more collagen than those in glucose at a physiological concentration. Amino acid analysis of the extracted collagen demonstrated twice as much hydroxyproline in each sample of the high glucose medium. Isotope incorporation studies confirmed that incubation in a medium equivalent to a plasma glucose level of 300 *milligrams* percent does result in increased collagen synthesis.

From the previous discussion, it can be concluded that increased synthesis plays a central role in the excessive accumulation of glomerular basement membrane in the diabetic kidney. While decreased degradation may also occur in diabetes, direct evidence for this is currently lacking. The findings of decreased glomerular *beta*-glycosidase activities (Chang, 1976; Fushima and Tarui, 1976) and urinary glomerular basement membrane-like protein (Weil, Nozawa, Koss, Weber, Reemtsma, and McIntosh, 1976) in diabetic rats, however, have prompted speculation that decreased glycoprotein catabolism may, in fact, play a role in basement membrane accumulation. Since increased glycosylation may also reduce the susceptibility of glycoproteins to proteolysis (Birkeland and Christensen, 1975), increased synthesis or decreased catabolism of the disaccharide units may also influence the degradation of basement membrane peptides. The elevation of serum protease inhibitors associated with diabetes might also be a contributing factor in this process (Brownlee, 1976).

CONCLUSIONS

The biochemical studies discussed in this review have clearly shown that increased synthesis of glomerular basement membrane occurs in the diabetic state. Furthermore, it seems probable that there is also a relatively greater production of basement membrane components which contain collagen-like units rich in hydroxylysine-linked disaccharide. Differential subunit incorporation studies in progress in several laboratories should help to answer this question. This increased synthesis, perhaps in conjunction with decreased degradation, would ultimately result in capillary occlusion and glomerular hyalinization. Alterations in basement membrane composition could well play a role in the increased permeability of the glomerular filtration barrier, leading to the continuous, nonselective and irreversible proteinuria which, together with the decreasing GFR, characterizes diabetic nephropathy. Insulin deficiency and its associated changes in metabolites and hormones may affect specific steps in the biosynthesis of basement membrane directly or via less specific glomerular cell injury. Although the sequence leading from the diabetic state to the resultant glomerular basement membrane changes remains conjectural at present, the focal character of diabetic glomerular disease suggests that both regional cell injury and systemic metabolic abnormalities are involved in the pathogenesis of these lesions. It is hoped that a fuller understanding of the mechanisms involved in the pathogenesis of the diabetic glomerular basement membrane changes will lead to the development of effective therapeutic modalities (Maragoudakis, Kalinsky, and Wasvary, 1978).

REFERENCES

Beisswenger, P. 1973. Specificity of the chemical alteration in the diabetic glomerular basement membrane. *Diabetes* 22:744-750.

Beisswenger, P.J. 1976. Glomerular basement membrane: Biosynthesis and chemical composition in the streptozocin diabetic rat. *J. Clin. Invest.* **58**:844-852.

Beisswenger, P.J. and Spiro, R.G. 1970. Human glomerular basement membrane: Chemical alteration in diabetes mellitus. *Science* **168**:596-598.

Beisswenger, P.J. and Spiro, R.G. 1973. Studies on the human glomerular basement membrane: Composition, nature of the carbohydrate units and chemical changes in diabetes. *Diabetes* 22:180-193.

Birkeland, A.J. and Christensen, T.B. 1975. Resistance of glycoproteins to proteolysis: Ribonuclease A and B compared. *J. Carb. Nucl.* **2**:83-90.

Brownlee, M. 1976. *Alpha*-2 macroglobulin and reduced basement membrane degradation in diabetes. *Lancet* **1**:779-780.

Brownlee, M. and Cahill, G.F. 1979. Diabetic control and vascular complication. pp. 29-70. **IN** R. Paoletti and A.M. Gotto (Eds.) *Atherosclerosis Reviews*. Vol. 4. New York: Raven Press

Brownlee, M. and Spiro, R.G. 1979. Glomerular basement membrane metabolism in the diabetic rat: *In vivo* studies. *Diabetes* 28:121-125.

Butcher, D., Kikkawa, R., Klein, L., and Miller, M. 1977. Size and weight of glomeruli isolated from human diabetic and nondiabetic kidneys. *J. Lab. Clin. Med.* **89**:544-555.

Chang, A.Y. 1976. Reduction of kidney *beta*-galactosidase in hereditary diabetic Chinese hamsters. *9th Congr. Int. Diab. Fed. ICS* 400:149. (Abstr.)

Cohen, M.P. and Khalifa, A. 1977. Effect of diabetes and insulin on rat renal glomerular protocollagen hydroxylase activities. *Biochim. Biophys. Acta* **496**:88-94.

Cohen, M.P. and Klein, C.V. 1976. Evidence for heterogeneous origin of glomerular basement membrane. *Biochem. Biophys. Res. Commun.* 77:1326-1332.

Cohen, M.P. and Klein, C.V. 1979. Glomerulopathy in rats with diabetes. Accumulation of glomerular basement membrane analogous to human diabetic nephropathy. *J. Exp. Med.* **149**:623-631.

Cohen, M.P. and Vogt, C.A. 1972. Evidence for enhanced basement membrane synthesis and lysine hydroxylation in renal glomerulus in experimental diabetes. *Biochem. Biophys. Res. Commun.* **49**:1542-1546.

Cohen, M.P. and Vogt, C.A. 1975a. Collagen synthesis and secretion by isolated rat renal glomeruli. *Biochim. Biophys. Acta* **393**:78-87.

Cohen, M.P. and Vogt, C.A. 1975b. The effect of diabetes on renal lysine utilization. *Horm. Metab. Res.* **7**:338-342.

DeOlivera, M.H. 1976. Membrana basal glomerular: Estudo bioquimico da membrana basal glomerular normal e suas variacoes com a idade e com a diabetes mellitus. Doctoral thesis.

Fox, C.J. and Darby, S.C. 1977. Blood glucose control and glomerular capillary basement membrane thickening in experimental diabetes. *Brit. Med. J.* **2**:605-607.

Freytag, J.W., Ohno, M., and Hudson, B.G. 1976. Bovine renal glomerular basement membrane: Assessment of proteolysis during isolation. *Biochem. Biophys. Res. Commun.* **72**:796-802.

Fushimi, H. and Tarui, S. 1976. *Beta*-glycosidases and diabetic microangiopathy. I. Decreases of *beta*-glycosidase activities in diabetic rat kidney. *J. Biochem.* **79**:265-270.

Grant, M.E., Harwood, R., and Williams, I.F. 1975. The biosynthesis of basement membrane collagen by isolated rat glomeruli. *Eur. J. Biochem.* **54**:531-540.

Grant, M.E., Harwood, R., and Williams, I.F. 1976. Increased synthesis of glomerular basement membrane collagen in streptozotocin diabetes. *J. Physiol.* **257**:56-57.

Gundersen, H.J.G. and Osterby, R. 1977. Glomerular size and structure in diabetes mellitus. II. Late abnormalities. *Diabetologia* **13**:43-48.

Hoyer, J.R. and Spiro, R.G. 1978. Studies on the rat glomerular basement membrane: Age-related changes in composition. *Arch. Biochem. Biophys.* **185**:496-503.

Hudson, B.G. and Spiro, R.G. 1972a. Studies on the native and reduced alkylated renal glomerular basement membrane: Solubility, subunit size, and reaction with cyanogen bromide. *J. Biol. Chem.* **247**:4229-4238.

Hudson, B.G. and Spiro, R.G. 1972b. Fractionation of glycoprotein components of the reduced alkylated renal glomerular basement membrane. *J. Biol. Chem.* **247**:4239-4247.

Kefalides, N.A. 1974. Biochemical properties of human glomerular basement membrane in normal and diabetic kidneys. *J. Clin. Invest.* **53**:403-407.

Khalifa, A. and Cohen, M.P. 1975. Glomerular protocollagen lysylhydroxylase activity in streptozotocin diabetes. *Biochim. Biophys. Acta* **386**:332-339.

Klein, L., Yoshida, M., and Miller, M. 1977. Does experimental diabetes in rats produce basement membrane thickening in renal glomeruli? *Diabetes* **26**:361.

Lazarow, A. and Speidel, E. 1964. The chemical composition of the glomerular basement membrane and its relationship to the production of diabetic complications. p. 127. **IN** M.D. Siperstein, A.R. Colwell, Sr., and K. Meyer (Eds.) *Small blood vessel involvement in diabetes mellitus*. Washington, DC: American Institute of Biological Sciences.

Maragoudakis, M., Kalinsky, H.J., and Wasvary, J. 1978. Effects of L-dopa, GPA 1734 and other agents on basement membrane biosynthesis. *J. Pharm. Exp. Ther.* **204**:377-383.

Osterby, R. 1978. Growth hormone enhances basement membrane thickening in experimental diabetes. *Diabetologia* **15**:487-489.

Peterson, D.T., Greene, W.C., and Reaven, G.M. 1971. Effects of experimental diabetes mellitus on kidney ribosomal protein synthesis. *Diabetes* **20**:649-654.

Price, R.G. Personal communication.

Price, R.G. and Spiro, R.G. 1977. Studies on the metabolism of the renal glomerular basement membrane: Turnover measurements in the rat with the use of radiolabeled amino acids. *J. Biol. Chem.* 252:8597-8602.

Rasio, E. and Bendayan, M. 1978. Le metabolisme de tissu capillaire et ses anomalies au cours du diabete. *Diab. Metab.* 4:57-62.

Reid, K.B.M. 1974. A collagen-like amino acid sequence in a polypeptide chain of human Clq (a subcomponent of the first component of complement). *Biochem. J.* **141**:189.

Risteli, J., Koivisto, V.A., Akerblom, H.K., and Kivirriko, K. (1976. Intracellular enzymes of collagen biosynthesis in rat kidney in streptozotocin diabetes. *Diabetes* **25**:1066-1070.

Sato, T. and Spiro, R.G. 1976. Studies on the subunit composition of the renal glomerular basement membrane. *J. Biol. Chem.* 251:4062-4070.

Seyer-Hansen, K. 1977. Renal hypertrophy in experimental diabetes: Relation to severity of diabetes. *Diabetologia* **13**:141-143.

Spiro, R.G. 1967a. Studies on the renal glomerular basement membrane: Preparation and chemical composition. *J. Biol. Chem.* 242:1915-1922.

Spiro, R.G. 1967b. Studies on the renal glomerular basement membrane: Nature of the carbohydrate units and their attachment to the peptide portion. *J. Biol. Chem.* **242**:1923-1932.

Spiro, R.G. 1971. Glycoproteins and diabetic microangiopathy. pp. 146-156. **IN** A. Marble, P. White, and R.F. Bradley (Eds.) *Joslin's diabetes mellitus*. Philadelphia:

Spiro, R.G. 1973a. Glycoproteins. *Adv. Protein Chem.* 27:349-467.

Spiro, R.G. 1973b. Biochemistry of the renal glomerular basement membrane and its alterations in diabetes mellitus. *New Eng. J. Med.* **288**:1337-1342.

Spiro, R.G. 1976. Search for a biochemical basis of diabetic microangiopathy. *Diabetologia* **12**:1-14.

Spiro, R.G. and Spiro, M.J. 1971a. Effect of diabetes on the biosynthesis of the renal glomerular basement membrane: Studies on the glycosyltransferase. *Diabetes* **20**:641-648.

Spiro, R.G. and Spiro, M.J. 1971b. Studies on the biosynthesis of the hydroxylysine-linked disaccharide unit of basement membranes and collagens. I. Kidney glucosyltransferase. *J. Biol. Chem.* **246**:4899-4909.

Spiro, R.G. and Spiro, M.J. 1971c. Studies on the biosynthesis of the hydroxylysine-linked disaccharide unit of basement membranes and collagens. II. Kidney galactosyltransferase. *J. Biol. Chem.* **246**:4910-4918.

Taylor, S.A. and Price, R.G. 1977. Characterization of subunits of rat glomerular basement membrane. *Biochem. Soc. Trans.* **5**:236-238.

Villee, D.B. and Lowers, M.L. 1977. Effect of glucose and insulin on collagen secretion by human skin fibroblasts *in vitro*. *Nature* **268**:156-158.

Weil, R., Nozawa, M., Koss, M., Weber, C., Reemtsma, K., and McIntosh, R. 1976. The kidney in streptozotocin diabetic rats. Morphologic, ultrastructural, and function studies. *Arch. Pathol. Lab. Med.* **100**:37-49.

Westberg, A.G. and Michael, A.F. 1970. Human glomerular basement membrane: Preparation and composition. *Biochemistry* **9**:3837-3846.

Westberg, A.G. and Michael, A.F. 1973. Human glomerular basement membrane: Chemical composition in diabetes mellitus. *Acta Med. Scand.* **194**:39-47.

Yagihashi, S., Goto, Y., Kakizaki, M., and Kaseda, N. 1978. Thickening of glomerular basement membrane in spontaneously diabetic rats. *Diabetologia* **15**:309-313.

DIABETIC GLOMERULOPATHY: A DYNAMIC PROCESS PRODUCED BY THE DIABETIC ENVIRONMENT

M.W. Steffes, D.M. Brown, and S.M. Mauer

Departments of Laboratory Medicine and Pathology
and Pediatrics
University of Minnesota Medical School
Minneapolis, MN 55455

INTRODUCTION

Renal lesions constitute a major factor in the morbidity and mortality of diabetes mellitus; however, the mechanisms underlying the development of diabetic glomerulopathy remain obscure. As a result, the efficacy of current medical management in affecting the development of renal disease in the diabetic population has not been conclusively determined. The central question considers whether diabetic vascular disease exists prior to clinical onset of diabetes or develops solely in relation to the underlying metabolic derangement (Cahill, Etzwiler, and Freinkel, 1976; Siperstein, Foster, Knowles, Levine, Madison, and Roth, 1977). Evidence emphasizing the need to initiate careful control of diabetes in order to alter the development of diabetic glomerulopathy arises from experiments in animals and observations made in man.

EXPERIMENTS IN ANIMALS

Rats, rendered diabetic by administration of streptozotocin (65 *mg/kg*) have plasma glucose levels that are significantly higher, and insulin values that are significantly lower, than those measured in age-matched normal controls. Intravenous glucose tolerance tests at six months following induction of diabetes reflect a marked difference between normal and diabetic animals in their ability to clear a glucose load. Similarly, the insulin re-

---

Supported by grants from the National Institute of Health (AM-17697) and the American Diabetes Association, Minnesota Affiliate.

sponse in the diabetic animals is markedly blunted as compared to control rats (Steffes, Sutherland, Mauer, Leonard, Najarian, and Brown, 1975).

The diabetic rat develops renal lesions not unlike those documented in man. The glomerular basement membrane increases significantly in thickness in diabetic as compared to control animals (Hägg, 1975). By grading the thickness of the glomerular mesangium, differences between normal and diabetic kidneys can be demonstrated, with the diabetic kidney possessing an increased mesangial matrix at six months of diabetes (Mauer, Michael, Fish, and Brown, 1975; Mauer, Sutherland, Steffes, Leonard, Najarian, Michael, and Brown, 1974). The mesangial matrix alterations demonstrated with the light microscope are focal in nature, although aggregate differences between diabetic and normal kidneys are readily perceived (Figure 1). A more uniform alteration observed in the diabetic glomerulus is the deposition of immunoglobulins in the mesangium (Mauer *et al.*, 1974). The specificity of these lesions for diabetes has been underlined by experiments in which kidneys were transplanted from normal to diabetic, inbred rats (Lee, Mauer, Brown, Sutherland, Michael, and Najarian, 1974). Within two months of transplantation, mesangial changes of diabetes appeared in the previously normal kidney, eliminating the diabetogenic agent as a cause of the nephropathy.

Islet transplantation experimentally tests the efficacy of control, or reversibility, of the diabetic state in affecting diabetic glomerulopathy. Using the method of Leonard, Lazarow, and Hegre (1973), islet transplantation returns glucose and insulin levels in previously diabetic rats to normal levels within three weeks while, over a longer period of time, the weight of the rats approaches that of the age-matched controls (Figure 2). Intravenous glucose tolerance tests in transplanted rats are essentially identical to those performed in normal animals, but markedly different from those in diabetic rats (Steffes *et al.*, 1975).

Pre- and posttransplant renal biopsies may be obtained to evaluate

---

Figure 1. Glomeruli from normal and diabetic rats prior to and following islet transplantation. (PAS stain)

a. Glomerulus from a diabetic rat prior to transplantation demonstrating thickened mesangial matrix and arteriolar narrowing.

b. Glomerulus from same rat as in Fig. 1a, three months after transplantation showing a decrease in mesangial matrix thickening.

c. Glomerulus from normal control rat at the three-month time period.

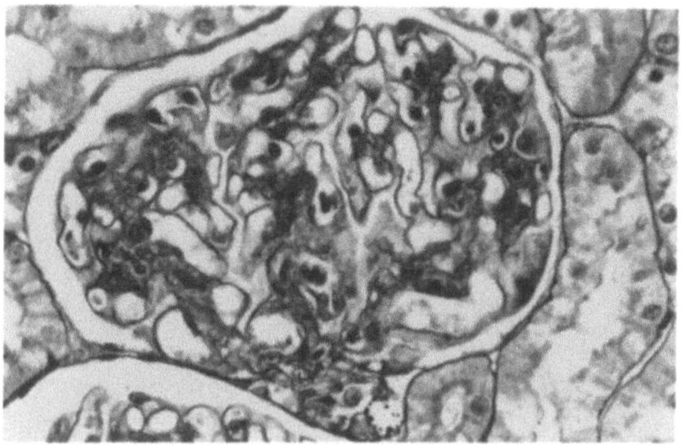

Figure 1a

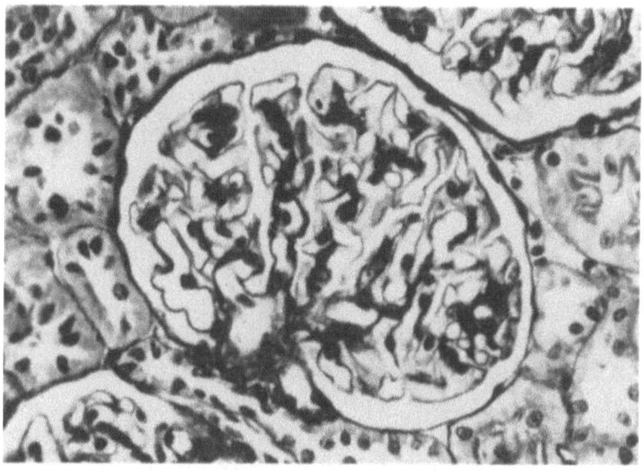

Figure 1b

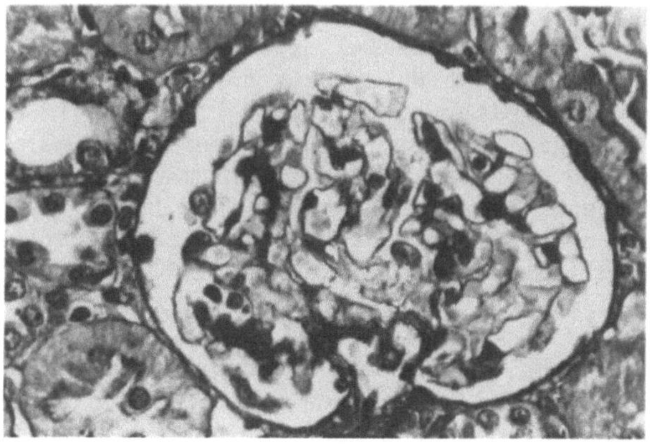

Figure 1c

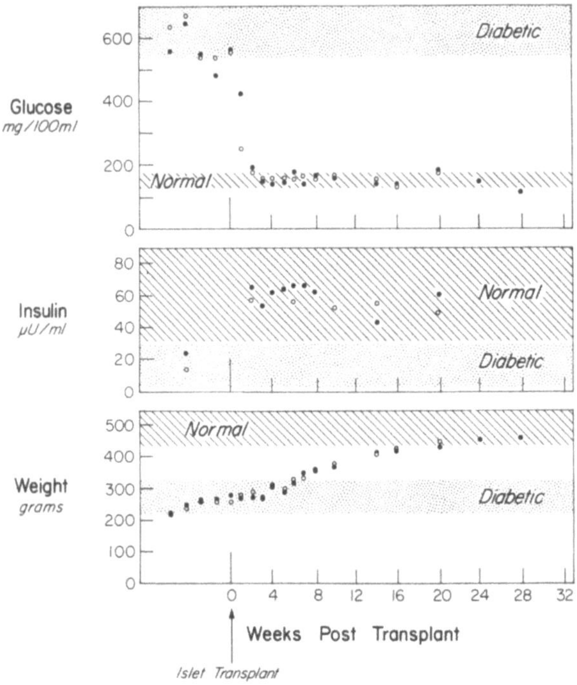

Figure 2. Individual plasma glucose and insulin levels and weights in two diabetic rats receiving transplanted islets. Pretransplant values were obtained from one week to four months prior to administration of islets. The values at the arrows were taken on the day of transplantation. The values for the individual animals are designated by either an open or closed circle.

the effect of islet transplantation and subsequent correction of plasma glucose and insulin levels on the renal lesions of diabetes in rats. The increased mesangial matrix either fails to progress, as it does in diabetic controls, or actually diminishes in amount following islet transplantation (Figure 1). A rapid and dramatic reduction in mesangial deposition of immunoglobulins occurs as soon as one to two weeks following islet transplantation (Mauer, Steffes, Sutherland, Najarian, Michael, and Brown, 1975). These results suggest that diabetic nephropathy in the rat is a dynamic and, at least during the time period studied, reversible process following amelioration of diabetes.

Using a dog model, Engerman, Bloodworth, Jr., and Nelson, (1977) recently reported the effect of improved diabetic control on the development of diabetic microangiopathy, specifically the prevention of the retinal lesions. They demonstrated a progression of retinopathy with time following induction of diabetes. In animals given excellent diabetic control, the retinopathy developed in a significantly reduced manner as compared to animals receiving poor control, findings compatible with the observations made in rats.

The metabolic derangements due to diabetes significantly affect the development of the secondary renal microangiopathy, probably by several mechanisms. Renal hypertrophy occurs within the first week of experimental diabetes in rats (Ross and Goldman, 1971; Seyer-Hansen, 1976, 1977), and the process continues for a longer period of time as a hyperplastic and hypertrophic response. When evaluated with respect to plasma glucose levels, the renal hypertrophy correlates with the elevated glucose values (Seyer-Hansen, 1977). In man the hypertrophy in early diabetes parallels an elevated glomerular filtration rate (Mogensen and Andersen, 1975) and an increase in glomerular volume (Østerby and Gundersen, 1975).

Uninephrectomy in the rat increases renal weight with and without diabetes (Ross and Goldman, 1971) and on a per nephron basis elevates glomerular filtration rate (Steffes, Brown, and Mauer, 1978) without changing blood pressure levels. Uninephrectomy in the diabetic rat accelerates the development of diabetic glomerulopathy. As soon as three months following nephrectomy, diabetic rats with uninephrectomy demonstrate enhanced thickening of the mesangial matrix and an increased deposition of immunoglobulins (Steffes *et al.*, 1978). Similarly, in rats with unilateral clipping of the renal artery (Goldblatt hypertension model), diabetic glomerulopathy develops more extensively on the unclipped (or unprotected) side, whereas the kidney with the clip demonstrates only minimal alterations due to diabetes (Mauer, Steffes, Azar, Sandberg, and Brown, 1978). These experiments suggest that diabetic microvascular lesions develop in an altered metabolic environment by a process that is enhanced by increased vascular flow.

OBSERVATIONS IN MAN

As alluded to above, increases in renal size, glomerular filtration rate, and filtration fraction occur prior to treatment in newly diagnosed patients with insulin-dependent diabetes (Mogensen, 1976). In patients with diabetes of long duration yet with no demonstrable proteinuria, glomerular filtration rate and renal plasma flow remain elevated (Mogensen, 1972). By utilizing a sensitive radioimmunoassay for albumin in the urine, Mogensen demonstrated in the newly diagnosed diabetic patient an increased excretion of albumin with exercise (Mogensen, 1976; Mogensen, and Vittinghus, 1975), a phenomenon perhaps related to the increased filtration fraction.

A series of observations by Mogensen of kidney weight, glomerular filtration rate, filtration fraction, and urinary albumin excretion underline the effect of control on the functional alterations of diabetes mellitus. The elevated levels of each of the parameters listed above returned toward normal levels following institution of appropriate medical management with insulin (Mogensen, 1976). The relation of these altered parameters of renal function and the eventual progression of diabetic glomerulopathy remains to be determined; however, the observations made in uninephrectomized rats (Steffes *et al.*, 1978) suggest that in increased glomerular filtration rate (and probably elevated renal plasma flow and glomerular capillary pressure) enchance the development of diabetic glomerulopathy.

Morphologic changes such as an increase in glomerular volume demonstrated in rats (Seyer-Hansen, 1976) also occur soon after onset of diabetes in man and may explain the physiologic changes outlined above. The increase in measured diameter (and thus volume) in glomeruli from diabetic subjects has been documented in people with diabetes of recent onset (Kroustrup, Gundersen, and Østerby, 1977; Østerby and Gundersen, 1975), and in patients with diabetes of long duration (Gundersen and Østerby, 1977). Butcher, Kikkawa, Klein, and Miller (1977) using sieving techniques, confirmed the work of Gundersen and Østerby by demonstrating increased glomerular size in patients with diabetes of short or long duration. The enlarged glomeruli from patients with diabetes of recent onset also demonstrated a significantly increased glomerular filtration surface (Kroustrup *et al.*, 1977). The enlarged filter provides a substantially enhanced surface area for glomerular filtration, but also, even without measurable increases in basement membrane thickness, implies a substantial increase in the mass of basement membrane.

Other morphologic changes defining diabetic microangiopathy and glomerulopathy occur early following onset of insulin-dependent diabetes mellitus. Mauer and his colleagues (Mauer, Barbosa, Vernier, Kjellstrand, Buselmeier, Simmons, Najarian, and Goetz, 1976; Mauer, Miller, Goetz, Barbosa, Simmons, Najarian, and Michael, 1976) examined by light and immunofluorescent microscopy the changes due to diabetes in normal kidneys transplanted to diabetic recipients. Within two years following transplantation they observed, in the grafted kidney, arteriolar hyalinosis and increased immunofluorescent staining of renal extracellular membranes, changes due to and reflecting diabetes in the recipient. Westberg and Michael (1972) in reviewing kidneys from children with diabetes, found glomerular basement membrane staining for IgG and other proteins within four years after the onset of disease. Since they were unable to obtain tissue from patients with diabetes of less than four years' duration, the lesions observed may occur even sooner after onset of diabetes.

The thickness of the glomerular basement membrane also reflects the progression of diabetic microangiopathy (Siperstein *et al.*, 1977). As referenced above, an increase in basement membrane thickness occurs in diabetic rats (Hägg, 1974), an observation which we have recently confirmed (Steffes, Brown, and Mauer, unpublished results). In man, glomerular basement membrane thickening occurs early after the onset of diabetes (Østerby, 1975) and it progresses with duration. The newly reported observations of an increase in surface area, when matched to the documented enhanced thickness of the basement membrane, suggest profound alterations in basement membrane synthesis and/or degradation soon after the initiation of insulin-dependent diabetes mellitus.

Finally, a clinical correlate to the enhanced plasma flow experiments (uninephrectomy and Goldblatt hypertension) also indicates a role of renal flow and/or pressure in the development of diabetic microangiopathy (Berkman and Rifkin, 1973). A patient with adult-onset diabetes and unilateral arteriosclerotic occlusion of the renal artery was studied. As with experimental diabetes, the kidney with the occluded artery had few pathologic changes characteristic of diabetes, whereas the hypertrophied, unprotected kidney contained enlarged glomeruli with thickened mesangial areas and nodular diabetic glomerulosclerosis. Although documentation was unobtainable, one might speculate that the increased flow to the hypertrophied kidney served to accelerate the development of diabetic microangiopathy.

COMPARISONS--MAN AND ANIMALS

Experimental diabetic glomerulopathy in rats does not resemble that in man in every morphologic and temporal aspect; however, it provides a system within which the functional and morphologic alterations may be characterized and compared. Thus, the glomerulus from a patient with diabetes or a rat with experimental diabetes enlarges in total size very soon after onset (Østerby and Gundersen, 1975; Seyer-Hansen, 1976). Also, it contains increased amounts of mesangial components (Iidaka, McCoy, and Kimmelstiel, 1968; Mauer *et al.*, 1972), thickened glomerular basement membranes (Hagg, 1974; Østerby, 1975; Steffes *et al.*, unpublished results), and abnormal deposits of immunoglobulins in the mesangium (Mauer *et al.*, 1976; Westberg and Michael, 1972). These similarities in morphologic changes in diabetes may reflect underlying pathologic processes common to diabetes mellitus of any etiology.

The observations made in man and animals demonstrating accelerated development of diabetic glomerulopathy in relation to increased flow and pressure (Berkman and Rifkin, 1973; Mauer *et al.*,

1978; Steffes *et al.*, 1978) strongly suggest that vascular alterations in diabetes affect the development of the lesions. Ditzel (1976), in discussing the significance of oxygen transport impairment in diabetes, suggested a compensatory increase in vascular flow to provide a normal capacity to deliver oxygen. Additionally, he has postulated that the enhanced local flow causes diabetic microangiopathy. In animals and man it is clear that vascular flow influences the development of diabetic microangiopathy. The pathophysiologic basis of diabetic angiopathy remains to be defined; however, delineation of factors affecting the process may permit medical management of microangiopathy even when control of the underlying diabetic disorder remains elusive.

REFERENCES

Berkman, J. and Rifkin, H. 1973. Unilateral nodular diabetic glomerulosclerosis (Kimmelstiel-Wilson): Report of a case. *Metabolism* **22**:715-722.

Butcher, D., Kikkawa, R., Klein, L., and Miller, M. 1977. Size and weight of glomeruli isolated from human diabetic and non-diabetic kidneys. *J. Lab. Clin. Med.* **89**:544-553.

Cahill, G.F. Jr., Etzwiler, D.D., and Freinkel, N. 1976. Blood glucose control in diabetes. *Diabetes* **25**:237-239.

Ditzel, J. 1976. Oxygen transport impairment in diabetes. *Diabetes* **25**:832-838.

Engerman, R., Bloodworth, J.M. Jr., and Nelson, S. 1977. Relationship of microvascular disease in diabetes to metabolic control. *Diabetes* **26**:760-769.

Gundersen, H.J.G. and Østerby, R. 1977. Glomerular size and structure in diabetes mellitus. II. Late abnormalities. *Diabetologia* **13**:43-48.

Hägg, E. 1974. Glomerular basement membrane thickening in rats with long-term diabetes. A quantitative electron microscopic study. *Acta. Path. Microbiol. Scand.* Sec. A. **82**:211-219.

Iidaka, K., McCoy, J., and Kimmelstiel, P. 1968. The glomerular mesangium. A quantitative analysis. *Lab. Invest.* **19**:573-579.

Kroustrup, J.P., Gundersen, H.J.G., and Østerby, R. 1977. Glomerular size and structure in diabetes mellitus. III. Early enlargement of the capillary surface. *Diabetologia* **13**:207-210.

Lee, C.S., Mauer, S.M., Brown, D.M., Sutherland, D.E.R., Michael, A.F., and Najarian, J.S. 1974. Renal transplantation in diabetes mellitus in rats. *J. Exp. Med.* **139**:793-800.

Leonard, R.J., Lazarow, A., and Hegre, O.D. 1973. Pancreatic islet transplantation in the rat. *Diabetes* **22**:413-438.

Mauer, S.M., Barbosa, J., Vernier, R.L., Kjellstrand, C.M., Buselmeier, T.J., Simmons, R.L., Najarian, J.S., and Goetz, F.C. 1976. Development of diabetic vascular lesions in normal kidneys transplanted into patients with diabetes mellitus. *N. Eng. J. Med.* **295**:916-920.

Mauer, S.M., Miller, K., Goetz, F.C., Barbosa, J., Simmons, R.L., Najarian, J.S., and Michael, A.F. 1976. Immunopathology of renal extracellular membranes in kidneys transplanted into patients with diabetes mellitus. *Diabetes* **25**:709-712.

Mauer, S.M., Steffes, M.W., Azar, S., Sandberg, S.K., and Brown, D.M. 1978. The effects of Goldblatt hypertension on the development of glomerular lesions of diabetes mellitus in the cat. *Diabetes* **27**:738-744.

Mauer, S.M., Steffes, M.W., Sutherland, D.E.R., Najarian, J.S., Michael, A.F., and Brown, D.M. 1975. Studies of the rate of regression of the glomerular lesions in diabetic rats treated with pancreatic islet transplantation. *Diabetes* **24**:280-285.

Mauer, S.M., Sutherland, D.E.R., Steffes, M.W., Leonard, R.J., Najarian, J.S., Michael, A.F., and Brown, D.M. 1974. Pancreatic islet transplantation: Effects on the glomerular lesions of experimental diabetes in the rat. *Diabetes* **23**:748-753.

Mogensen, C.E. 1972. Glomerular filtration rate and renal plasma flow in long-term juvenile diabetics without proteinuria. *Brit. Med. J.* 4:257-259.

Mogensen, C.E. 1976. Renal function changes in diabetes. *Diabetes* **25**:872-879.

Mogensen, C.E. and Andersen, M.J.F. 1975. Increased kidney size and glomerular filtration rate in untreated juvenile diabetes: Normalization by insulin-treatment. *Diabetologia* **11**:221-224.

Mogensen, C.E. and Vittinghus, E. 1975. Urinary albumin excretion during exercise in juvenile diabetes. *Scand. J. Clin. Lab. Invest.* **35**:295-300.

Østerby, R. 1975. Early phases in the development of diabetic glomerulopathy. *Acta. Med. Scand. Suppl.* **574**:1-80.

Østerby, R. and Gundersen, H.J.G. 1975. Glomerular size and structure in diabetes mellitus. I. Early abnormalities. *Diabetologia* **11**:225-229.

Ross, J. and Goldman, J.K. 1971. Effect of streptozotocin-induced diabetes on kidney weight and compensatory hypertrophy in the rat. *Endocrinology* **88**:1079-1082.

Seyer-Hansen, K. 1976. Renal hypertrophy in streptozotocin-diabetic rats. *Clin. Sci. Mol. Med.* **51**:551-555.

Seyer-Hansen, K. 1977. Renal hypertrophy in experimental diabetes: Relation to severity of diabetes. *Diabetologia* **13**:141-143.

Siperstein, M.D., Foster, D.W., Knowles, H.C. Jr., Levine, R., Madison, L.L., and Roth, J. 1977. Control of blood glucose and diabetic vascular disease. *N. Eng. J. Med.* **296**:1060-1063.

Steffes, M.W., Brown, D.M., and Mauer, S.M. 1978. Diabetic glomerulopathy following nephrectomy in the rat. *Diabetes* **27**:35-41.

Steffes, M.W., Sutherland, D.E.R., Mauer, S.M., Leonard, R.J., Najarian, J.S., and Brown, D.M. 1975. Plasma insulin and glucose levels in diabetic rats prior to and following islet transplantation. *J. Lab. Clin. Med.* **85**:75-81.

Westberg, N.G. and Michael, A.F. 1972. Immunohistopathology of diabetic glomerulosclerosis. *Diabetes* **21**:163-174.

DISCUSSION FOLLOWING TALKS ON MICROVASCULAR COMPLICATIONS OF DIABETES MELLITUS

Dr. Guthrie

To open this discussion period, we have asked Dr. John Townsend, who is in the Department of Pathology here at the University of Missouri, to make a few comments regarding the colony of genetically diabetic animals that they have been following here in regard to vascular disease in these animals.

Dr. Townsend

I would like to take this opportunity to bring you up to date with regard to capillary basement membrane studies in the Department of Pathology colony of *Mystromys albicaudatus*. This South African rodent was brought into the United States in the early 1960's for experimental purposes and a few were brought to the University of Missouri in the late 1960's.

While observing the colony, it became apparent that there was excessive cage wetting. Subsequent studies demonstrated that many of the animals were hyperglycemic and glycosuric, and that some were also ketotic. This change was spontaneous and occurred in animals which were not obese.

A number of studies have subsequently been carried out to characterize the diabetic state in these animals (Goeken, Packer, Rose, and Stuhlman, 1972; Packer, Kraner, Rose, Stuhlman, and Nelson, 1970; Schmidt, Martin, Stuhlman, Townsend, Lucas, and Vorbeck, 1974; Schmidt, Martin, Townsend, and Vorbeck, 1977; Srivastava, Townsend, Stuhlman, and Lucas, 1974; Stuhlman, Packer, and Doyle, 1972; Stuhlman, Packer, Doyle, Brown, and Townsend, 1975; Stuhlman, Srivastava, Schmidt, Vorbeck, and Townsend, 1974). Currently, activity is under way to examine the animals for microangiopathy.

The first vessel changes related todiabetes were observed during examination of the kidneys by light microscopy (Riley, Stuhlman, Van Peenen, Esterly, and Townsend, 1975). These changes consisted of an increase in glomerular basement membrane and increase in mesangium.

Subsequently, examination of the rectus femoris muscle for capillary microangiopathy has revealed such changes in a pilot group of animals (Yesus, Esterly, Stuhlman, and Townsend, 1976) and a large-scale study is now in progress to characterize these changes. Preliminary indications are that we are dealing with a spontaneously diabetic animal that is not obese and has microvascular changes in renal glomeruli and skeletal muscle.

Mrs. Jan Franz has provided us with longstanding and excellent technical assistance and has been of great service to us in maintaining the colony of animals.

In conclusion, I would like to express our deep appreciation to Dr. Robert Jackson for his continued support. He has not only been a source of encouragement and advice, he has shared space in his facilities so that we can carry on certain aspects of this work.

Dr. Klachko

I have a question for Dr. Steffes. With the very nice demonstration of the immunofluorescence of the IgG in the glomeruli, obviously there is antibody deposition there. Some people have speculated that perhaps these are antibodies to exogenous insulin or associated proteins. However, I assume from the low weight of the streptozotocin-treated rats that they were not treated with insulin. Is that correct?

Dr. Steffes

Yes. The immunoglobulins have never been shown to fix complement, so we have felt that it is not an immunologic reaction. From other studies we have speculated that the mesangium clears exogenous components from the glomerulus. The IgG, C_3, and IgM are all proteins that, to a limited degree, normally pass through the mesangium during the filtration process. Somehow in the diabetic, the capability of clearing these proteins is diminished.

With respect to the process being due to streptozotocin, I will cite the work of Lee, Mauer, Brown, Sutherland, Michael, and Najarian (1974). Kidneys from normal rats transplanted to diabetic animals developed the same lesions as kidneys from diabetic rats. The transplanted kidneys were never exposed to streptozotocin; thus, we believe the changes shown result from the altered metabolic environment in diabetes and not from streptozotocin.

Dr. Guthrie

In view of the very low serum insulin levels of these diabetic rats, how do you keep them alive without insulin treatment?

Dr. Steffes

These diabetic rats--65 *mg/kg* is the dose of streptozotocin we give them--will exist with plasma glucose levels anywhere from 400-800 *mg/dl*. They'll live for nine, ten, or eleven months. They will be terrifically hyperphagic and they will take massive quantities of water, but they will exist.

I didn't bring any slides along to show you these animals. The first appearance that does occur after kidney transplantation is a clinical change. They look better and the fur is better.

Dr. Guthrie

I've seen those pictures, and those are pretty sick-looking rats before you do something to them.

Dr. Jackson, would you like to comment on the question that Dr. Steffes brought up regarding reversibility of the microvascular changes. Dr. Williamson also alluded to that.

Dr. Jackson

At the University of Missouri, we have observed a small group of seven postpubescent boys, all of whom have slightly increased capillary basement membrane thickness (CBMT) at the time of onset of overt diabetes. After their disease was maintained in a high degree of control for over seven months, the capillary basement membranes had thinned and were well within the mid-range for normal boys.

We are accumulating additional longitudinal data on our patients in late adolescence and early adult life. Although these data are limited, the findings have been consistent. Patients maintained in "good" control have not had increased CBMT, patients who have maintained a higher degree of control have had some decrease in CBMT, and all patients in lower degrees of control have had progressive increase in CBMT. We have not found a definitive increase in capillary basement membrane thickness in children with diabetes prior to puberty regardless of duration or degree of control of their disease. Before puberty, children in lower degrees of control have delayed linear growth and maturation. We were surprised to find that adolescent girls in lower degrees of control had increased CBMT earlier than boys of similar age and duration of diabetes. Last year Dr. Williamson, in collaboration with the pediatric staff at Washington University, confirmed our findings that increased thickening of the capillary basement membrane does not occur prior to puberty. Consequently, I would like to ask Dr. Williamson to speculate as to which other endocrine factors occurring during maturation might be responsible for the microvascular changes.

Also, I would like to know the sex of the triplets and additional clinical information concerning the age of onset and degree of control of the diabetes in the two siblings who developed overt diabetes. I ask this, inasmuch as the diabetic child with minimal CBMT had the disease for a longer period of time than the other with more advanced CBMT. In our experience it is easier to attain and maintain a higher degree of control when the onset of diabetes occurs before puberty. During mid- or late-adolescence, it usually is more difficult to attain good compliance.

Dr. Guthrie

Dr. Williamson, would you like to respond to these questions?

Dr. Williamson

Well, first regarding the triplets and twins, I should acknowledge that the twin's study was done by Dr. Gerich and his associates in San Francisco and John just reminds me that those were girls.

The triplets that we looked at with Dr. Soeldner and Dr. Gonda were males. The point that you raised about the time of onset in the relation to puberty in the two diabetic members of the triplets is an interesting one. It's perplexing but, I guess, not too surprising that the one with the diabetes of ten years' duration had less evidence of thickening than the one with three years of duration. They were 22 years old at the time we studied them.

And, although we know there could be a lot of variation in any group of diabetics you look at, it's interesting that at least in this case I think it would fit with your suggestion. The diabetic with ten years' duration did have his onset just right at the time of puberty or perhaps just before, whereas the one with the three-year duration was, obviously, postpubertal at the time of onset and the entire duration was postpubertal.

Your other question had to do with what this puberty-related factor might be. Of course, that's really open for speculation. It's intriguing to us that in normal subjects the rate of thickening through the puberty years and postpubertal years is essentially the same in both sexes. There is no significant sex difference. It's only between ages roughly 30 and 50 that there is a significant difference and then women catch up with men after the menopause. Well, these sorts of observations would suggest that sex hormones *per se* are not the critical factor because the basement membranes are increasing in thickness at essentially the same rate in young men and women. The fact that they increase so rapidly in postmenopausal women would suggest that if it's not sex hormones *per se*, maybe it has something to do with gonadotropins or some other pituitary or hypothalamic factor that hasn't really been identified. So this is where our thinking is, but we really don't know what the factor might be. I think if we could identify it, that would be a real advance.

Dr. Jackson

Thank you, Dr. Williamson. I hope this discussion will help stimulate some young investigators to find the answers to these serious questions.

Question

The postpubertal duration of disease makes the disease worse. It can increase thickening according to Dr. Williamson. Now, the correlation sometimes was .2 or .25; am I correct?

Dr. Williamson

I think it was .25 or .28.

Question

Isn't that a weak correlation?

Dr. Williamson

Well, it's not as strong as you might like, but it's certainly statistically significant in the group we looked at. Most people think this is a multifactorial disease, so the fact that we can demonstrate anything at all here is probably important; particularly if you compare that figure with the correlation between basement membrane thickness and the total duration of diabetes, which I didn't show, where there is absolutely no correlation.

Dr. Jackson

Another factor to take into consideration is the delay in maturation which invariably occurs in patients maintained in lower degrees of control. And, sad to say, this comprises the majority of children with overt diabetes. Consequently, we need to use maturational age rather than chronological age as the criterion for analysis.

Dr. Williamson

I should add to that that we were using an arbitrary age for onset of puberty rather than really knowing the exact onset of puberty in each subject which might have made the correlation a little stronger.

Dr. Jackson

Our observations indicate that accurate serial observations of linear growth and maturation are very important and, in our experience, only children in lower degrees of control by our criteria, have delayed growth and maturation.

Dr. Sanny

I was wondering if anybody would be willing to comment on the future feasibility of *beta* cell transplant in humans for diabetic control.

Dr. Guthrie

Dr. Steffes, would you like to comment on that?

Dr. Steffes

Well, while I'm not working with the surgeons at our place nearly as much as I used to, I have a pretty good idea of the kinds of things they're doing. I really believe that *beta* cell transplantation is going to work but, in terms of doing anything about diabetes for the population, it will not, because you are not going to be able to transplant that many people. The sources are limited and all the factors involved in any kind of transplantation currently are overwhelming in terms of trying to transplant a diabetic population.

It will certainly allow us to answer questions in people that now we can only answer in animals. I really believe it's going to work, but I think that, if we're going to do something for all diabetics, trying to treat each person in the best possible way will be more significant than transplantation.

Dr. Brownlee

I wanted to make one brief comment about a relatively new approach to this which Dr. Jean-Michel Dubernand from Lyon, France, is pioneering in. Essentially, he is transplanting cadaveric pancreas but he has overcome a major surgical technical problem which was exocrine proteolysis digesting the anastomosis site. What he simply has done is to inject the pancreatic duct with neoprine, a compound which polymerizes upon contact with acid. This essentially embalms the exocrine tissue while leaving the endocrine function intact. The organ can then be simply interposed (via its splenic vessels) between the external iliac artery and vein of the recipient. All of the cases he's done have been in patients undergoing simultaneous kidney transplantation. There has been no problem with the proteolytic breakdown of the anastomosis, so from a technical point-of-view, that seems to be a very encouraging thing.

In the series that he has presented there were several patients who had rejected their renal homografts despite increased immunosuppression, but throughout the whole course had maintained normal endocrine pancreatic function.

This may possibly be so because the concentration of transplantation antigens is said to be greater in renal cells than in endocrine pancreas. This, then, may be less of a requirement for immunosuppression with endocrine tissue than there would be for the kidneys. If these results are confirmed by further work, this would be a very intriguing kind of therapeutic approach, especially in certain extreme cases. The patients presented by Dr. Dubernand were doing quite well.

Dr. Guthrie

Nonetheless, I think for the next few years I will attempt to keep my diabetics under good control rather than await pancreas transplant. I think control certainly holds our best hope for diabetic patients at the moment.

Although transplant and other new developments are exciting and offer us possibilities for the future, the patient who is already blind and has severe glomerulosclerosis that is probably not reversible, is not going to benefit. The data that are becoming available that the severity of the vascular diseases are related to control makes it increasingly important to maintain control so that our patients are free of vascular disease or relatively so when the new developments do come along.

Certainly it is not possible to totally duplicate normal physiology, but the programs such as those that have been evolved over the years by a variety of people, including Dr. Jackson, can at least somewhat approximate normal physiology to the point that, as our data and that of others would tend to indicate, their diabetic patients do remain relatively free of vascular disease over a long period of time. And that can be done within a lifestyle which is acceptable to the patient. And I think that's important as well. There are a lot of things you could do to people to control their blood sugar that would not be acceptable to them within any kind of a liveable lifestyle. But programs which have been evolved by Dr. Jackson and others are certainly acceptable.

I just came here from Phoenix where I spoke to a group of osteopathic pediatricians from all over the country. And it was very gratifying that, since listening to an Audiodigest tape that I made a couple of years ago, they have adopted Dr. Jackson's methods of managing diabetes. And the gratifying thing was that their comments were, "It works; the patients feel better; they accept it; they like it; they like it better than the old methods of single-shot insulin therapy they were receiving; and they actually have a better life with fewer hypoglycemic reactions and a better ability to adapt into the culture in which they live." So the proof of the pudding, of course, is that these methods do work.

DISCUSSION REFERENCES

Goeken, J.A., Packer, J.T., Rose, S.D., and Stuhlman, R.A. 1972. Structure of the islets of Langerhans: Pathological studies in normal and diabetic *Mystromys albicaudatus*. *Arch. Path.* 93:123.

Lee, C.S., Mauer, S.M., Brown, D.M., Sutherland, D.E.R., Michael, A.J., and Najarian, J.S. 1974. Renal transplantation in diabetes mellitus in rats. *J. Exp. Med.* 139:793-800.

Packer, J.T., Kraner, K.L., Rose, S.D., Stuhlman, R.A., and Nelson, L.R. 1970. Diabetes mellitus in *Mystromys albicaudatus*. *Arch. Path.* **89**:410.

Riley, T., Stuhlman, R.A., Van Peenen, H.J., Esterly, J.A., and Townsend, J.F. 1975. Glomerular lesions of diabetes mellitus in *Mystromys albicaudatus*. *Arch. Path.* **99**:167.

Schmidt, G., Martin, A.P., Stuhlman, R.A., Townsend, J.F., Lucas, F.V., and Vorbeck. M.L. 1974. Evaluation of hepatic mitochondrial function in the spontaneously diabetic *Mystromys albicaudatus*. *Lab. Invest.* **30**:451.

Schmidt, G.E., Martin, A.P., Townsend, J.F., and Vorbeck, M.L. 1977. Basement membrane synthesis in spontaneously diabetic *Mystromys albicaudatus*. *J. Cell Biol.* **75**:155a.

Srivastava, P.K., Townsend, J.F., Stuhlman, R.A., and Lucas, F.V. 1974. Somatic chromosomes of the African white-tailed rat. *J. Heredity* **65**:223.

Stuhlman, R.A., Packer, J.T., and Doyle, R.E. 1972. Spontaneous diabetes mellitus in *Mystromys albicaudatus*: Repeated glucose values from 620 animals. *Diabetes* **21**:715.

Stuhlman, R.A., Packer, J.T., Doyle, R.E., Brown, R.V., and Townsend, J.F. 1975. Relationship between pancreatic lesions and serum glucose values in *Mystromys albicaudatus*. *Lab. Animal Sci.* **25**:168.

Stuhlman, R.A., Srivastava, P.K., Schmidt, G., Vorbeck, M.L., and Townsend, J.F. 1974. Characterization of diabetes mellitus in South African hamsters (*Mystromys albicaudatus*). *Diabetologia* **10**:685.

Yesus, Y.W., Esterly, J.A., Stuhlman, R.A., and Townsend, J.F. 1976. Significant muscle capillary basement membrane thickening in spontaneously diabetic *Mystromys albicaudatus*. *Diabetes* **25**:444.

DIABETES MELLITUS CHALLENGES FOR THE FUTURE

B.R. Boshell, M.D., and B.S. Trippe, M.D.

Diabetes Research and Education Hospital
Div. of Endocrinology
University of Alabama School of Medicine
Birmingham, AL 35294

OUTLINE

Introduction

Diagnosis of Diabetes mellitus

- Value of GTT
- New Criteria
- Genetic markers

Etiology of Diabetes mellitus

- Genetic
- Autoimmunity
- Obesity
  - receptors

Treatment

- General considerations
- Pancreatic transplantation
- Artificial pancreas
- Somatostatin and other compounds

Complications

- Sorbitol
- 2,3-DPG
- Control of various complications

Summary

INTRODUCTION

Diabetes mellitus remains an enigma in many ways in spite of the tremendous amount of research and writing that has occurred regarding this condition during the past 50 years. Nobel prizes have been awarded to Banting and Best (1922) for the discovery of insulin, Houssay (1937) for his pituitary investigations which spotlighted the extrapancreatic aspects of diabetes, to Sanger (1959) and colleagues for elucidating the amino acid structure of insulin, and to Sutherland and Rall (1958) for their classic studies in hormone action as manifest by changes in cyclic AMP.

In spite of these classical studies in diabetes that have received such widespread acclaim plus the exciting contributions of Yalow and Berson (1959) in developing the radioimmunoassay using insulin as a model and the important contribution of Steiner, Cunningham, Spigelman, and Aten (1967) in their pro-insulin studies, the exact answers to "What is Diabetes?" and "How does insulin work at the cellular level?" have not been found. Thus, we talk about a condition(s) that involves at least 5% of the population, doubles in incidence every 15 years, costs our economy six billion dollars per year, is the third leading cause of death, the most common cause of irreversible blindness, and the most important condition predisposing to accelerated vascular disease; yet, we are unsure as to what we are talking about. Considering the importance of diabetes and the impact that it makes each year on the health welfare of U.S. citizens alone, one is quite justified in suggesting that there are at least three more Nobel Prizes awaiting scientists in diabetic research: (1) the group that establishes concrete diagnostic tests for diabetes and elucidates the specific etiologies; (2) the group that discovers the mode of insulin action and *via* this develops more effective modes of therapy; and (3) the group that pinpoints the etiology and, hence, preventive methods for the complications of diabetes. These questions constitute challenges for the future.

One of the first challenges, however, is to establish adequate research funds to attract new scientists into the field of diabetes research. It is rather disconcerting to those interested in diabetes to note that as of 1975 there was only 43 million dollars allotted to diabetes research, as compared to 208 million dollars in heart research and 691 million dollars in cancer research. Significantly more money must be made available if research in diabetes is to prosper. The findings of the National Commission on Diabetes (Report of the National Commission on Diabetes to the Congress of the United States, submitted December 10, 1975) will, hopefully, stimulate an improvement in this regard.

DIAGNOSIS OF DIABETES MELLITUS

The diagnosis of diabetes is a difficult matter. Although we define diabetes as a relative or absolute deficiency of insulin, we are not quite sure that this is appropriate or all inclusive in that many factors suggest that diabetes, as we now know it, is a syndrome with heterogeneous expression, *i.e.*, biochemical, cellular, chromosomal, hormonal, etc. The classic oral glucose tolerance test which remains as our standard technique for the diagnosis of diabetes is affected by many factors (Chandalia and Boshell, 1970) and is considered by several authors to be arbitrary and inconclusive (Siperstein, 1976; Unger and Madison, 1958). Both clinicians and scientists continue their research for "The Holy Grail," a definitive absolute diagnostic test, or tests, for diabetes mellitus. A gaze into the past and a peek into the future bring forth some of the following possibilities: the synalbumin of Vallance-Owen (1964), the bound insulin of Antoniades (Antoniades, Gundersen, Beigelman, Pyle, and Bougas, 1962); the thickened capillary membrane of Siperstein (Siperstein, Norton, Unger, and Madison, 1966); the abnormal insulin of O'Brien (1970); the insulin deficiency and *beta* cell inertia as described by Yalow and Berson (1960); and the decreased insulin receptors of Roth (Archer, Gordon, and Roth, 1975). One must also think of the altered glucose receptors as described by Matschinsky (Matchinsky, Landgraf, Ellerman, and Kotler-Brajtburg, 1972)(Table 1). Perhaps we will eventually subclassify diabetes from the etiologic standpoint whereby we may in the future speak of specific kinds as manifested by particular defects or contributing causes as we now do with pneumonia. Only a few years ago the patient was thought of only as "a case of congestion" or pneumonia, whereas now specific bacteria, viruses, fungi, etc. can be identified as the offending agent and allow us to classify clearly and treat effectively. Many studies now suggest that basic etiologic differences exist in adult onset and juvenile diabetes. It will, of course, not be surprising if subclassification appears in both of these broad categories (Table 2).

Table 1. DIAGNOSTIC MARKERS OR TESTS FOR DIABETES MELLITUS

1.	Glucose tolerance test	
2.	Tolbutamide tolerance test	Unger & Madison
3.	Synalbumin	Vallance-Owen
4.	Bound insulin	Antoniades
5.	Thickened capillary membrane	Siperstein
6.	Abnormal insulin	O'Brien
7.	Insulin deficiency & *beta* cell inertia	Berson & Yalow
8.	Insulin receptors	Roth
9.	Glucose receptors	Matchinsky
10.	Specific genetic markers	Nerup
11.	Gene antibodies	Irvine

Table 2. *CLASSIFICATION OF DIABETES MELLITUS*

Futuristic
JUVENILE ONSET:
1. Viral
a. mumps
b. coxsackie$_{4,3,2,1}$
c. EMC
2. Simple autoimmune
3. Traumatic
4. Simple genetic
5. Miscellaneous
ADULT ONSET:
1. Simple genetic, *i.e.*, insulin deficiency
2. Tissue resistant
a. quantitative decrease in receptors
b. low receptor affinity
c. circulating receptor antibodies
3. Stress
a. hormonal
b. other
4. Miscellaneous

A strong familial appearance of diabetes in both juvenile onset and adult onset exists in spite of the fact that studies of identical twins (Tattersall and Pyke, 1972) suggest different modes of transmission of the two broad categories. One must not ignore the possibility that these two conditions may have an underlying similar genetic basis with different expressions caused by multiple environmental factors. Thus, theoretically, one might still search for the abnormal genes and, if located and isolated, introduce them into guinea pigs or other appropriate animals to produce antibodies that would allow us to identify the diabetes-prone fetus by doing an amniotic tap prior to birth and reacting this with the gene-specific antibody.

ETIOLOGY OF DIABETES MELLITUS

Genetic

The inability to have a controlled breeding program makes experiments and studies in human genetics very difficult. This complex problem is compounded when applied to diabetes mellitus because of the extremely varied way in which the diabetes may be expressed, *i.e.*, mild, moderate, severe, age of onset--early, middle, and late--mild chemical carbohydrate intolerance, overt disturbances in carbohydrate, fat and protein metabolism, full-blown ketoacidosis, hyperosmolar coma, etc. Animal models provide some insight into this problem. The inheritance of diabetes mellitus in the Chinese hamster has been shown to be determined by multiple alleles (Ganda and Soeldner, 1977). Even the animal studies, however, are complicated by the fact that dietary manipulations have a profound effect on the expression of carbohydrate intolerance (Wilkerson, Hyman, Kaufman, McCuistion, and Francis, 1960).

Reviews of both old and recent studies strongly suggest that the juvenile onset diabetic, *i.e.*, onset under the age of 40 years, differs from the adult onset in that identical twins both usually develop diabetes mellitus if one has the disorder in the adult onset group, whereas this occurs in less than 50% of the cases in the juvenile group (Gottlieb and Root, 1968; Tattersall and Pyke, 1972)(Table 3). These findings do not necessarily deny a similar genetic disorder in both groups but strongly suggest that environmental factors such as viral infections play a more important role in finalizing the overt expression of the disorder in the juvenile onset group (Table 4). The answer may be even simpler than this, however. Obesity is rampant, *i.e.*, about 80% (Williams and Porte, 1974) in the adult onset group and relatively rare in the juvenile onset group (White and Graham, 1971); therefore, it seems certain that a severe metabolic stress in the adult onset group may play a role in insuring the genetic expression of latent diabetes.

If multiple genes are involved, it may well be that juvenile

Table 3. GENETICS AND DIABETES

1. Identical twins	
a. Juvenile onset--concordance	<50%
b. Adult onset--concordance	100%
2. Offspring of conjugal diabetics	
overt diabetes	6-10%
chemical diabetes	25-40%
Estimate by age 85	
overt diabetes	33%
chemical diabetes	50%

Ganda & Soeldner

Table 4. VIRUSES AND DIABETES MELLITUS

		HISTORICAL
**1.	1899	Ketoacidosis following mumps (Harris)
**2.	1973	Diabetes mellitus and Coxsackie B_4 (Gamble & Taylor)
**3.	1971	Diabetes mellitus and congenital rubella (Forrest *et al.*)
*4.	1975	Encephalomyocarditis virus and juvenile onset diabetes mellitus (Craighead)
**5.	1974	Infectious mononucleosis (Burgess *et al.*)
**6.	1974	Infectious hepatitis (Adi)

* *animals*

** *humans*

diabetes is merely a form of adult onset disease, in that the juvenile onset type is only partially diabetic from the genotypic standpoint, whereas the adult onset group has the whole genetic orchestra essential to the development of diabetes. It appears that environmental factors, such as viruses, are necessary to produce the complete syndrome in the juvenile. The viral infection plus the subsequent reaction of the autoimmune system completely destroy the islets (Figure 1), producing insulin deficiency and insulin dependency, whereas the pure genetic syndrome, *i.e.*, adult onset diabetes, is milder and characterized by insulin resistance more so than insulin deficiency.

Future projects in evaluating the genetic influence in diabetes will involve more sophisticated tissue typing and epidemiological studies. Furthermore, answers may be found in more definitive evaluation of patients with chromosomal abnormalities in an attempt to identify the specific chromosomal locus of the genetic diabetic determinants. One must also consider the possibility that receptor proteins on the *beta* cell that bind glucose may be genetically controlled and be abnormal in the diabetic, thereby contributing to the etiology of this syndrome. More definitive genetic studies of the American Indians (Bennett, Burch, and Miller, 1971) and the Asians (Mimura, 1971) who have severe diabetes but a low incidence of ketoacidosis may be quite revealing.

Autoimmunity

The existence of HLA-linked diabetogenic genes can be theorized from prior work on immune response genes (Bach and van Rood, 1976a, 1976b, 1976c). Studies of the histocompatibility antigens

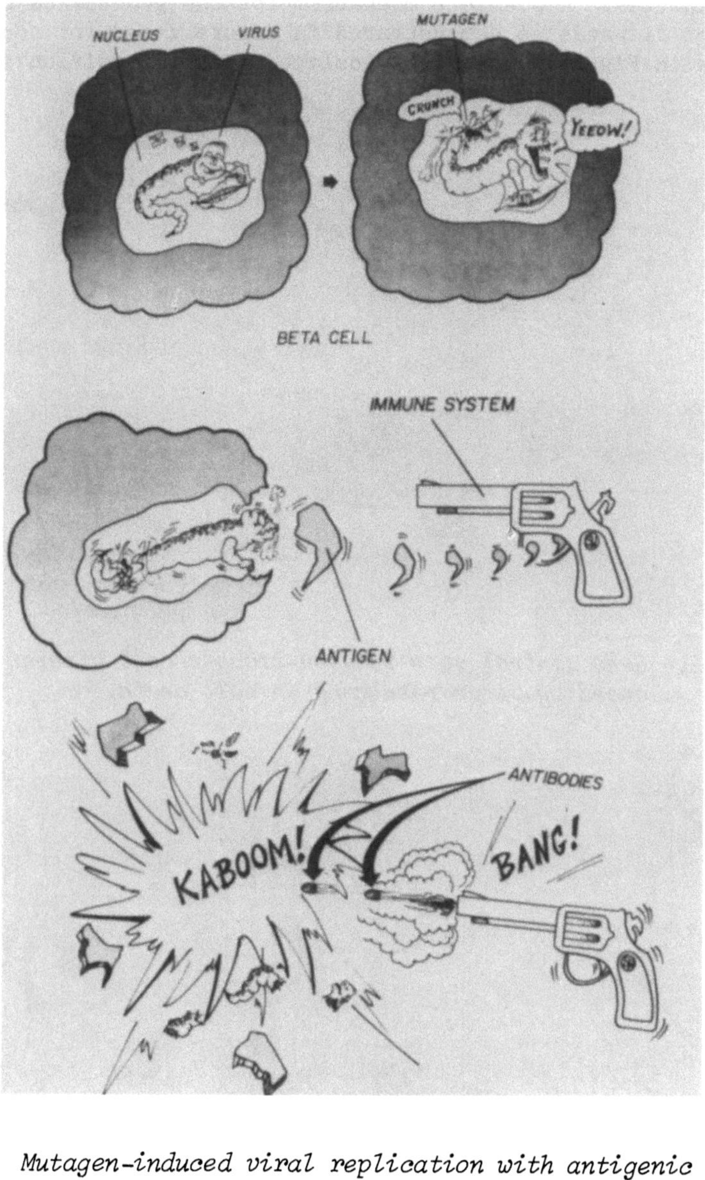

Figure 1. Mutagen-induced viral replication with antigenic stimulation causing immune system response and beta-cell destruction.

have suggested that a definite positive correlation of acute onset juvenile diabetes mellitus and HLA-8 and W15 antigens exist (Cudworth and Woodrow, 1975). This relationship is not found in adult onset diabetes. A possible mechanism for the generation of juvenile onset diabetes is demonstrated in Figure 2 and for adult onset diabetes in Figure 3. It is speculated that in addition to genes

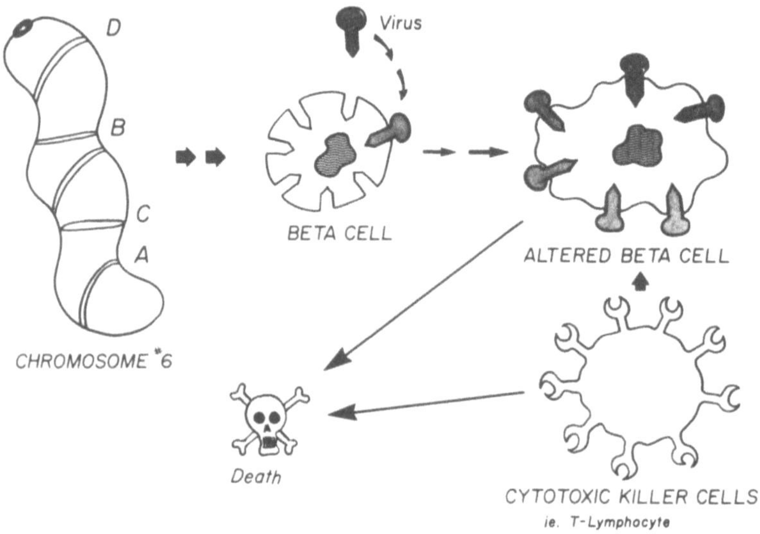

Figure 2. Gene control over insulin-trophic cell alteration induced by virus resulting in cell death.

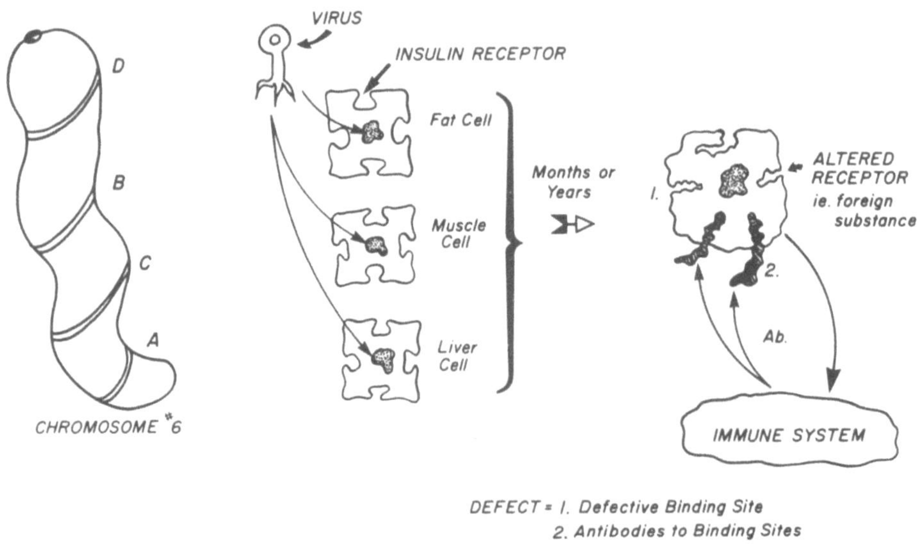

Figure 3. Multitargeted change in expression of diabetes with receptor alteration involving autoimmunity in the adult.

Table 5. DIABETES MELLITUS AND AUTOIMMUNE DISEASE

1. "Insulitis" in young diabetics dying shortly after diagnosis (Gepts)
2. Experimental "insulitis" produced by injection of homologous insulin (Renold) or homologous islet cell suspension (Nerup *et al.*)
3. Association of diabetes mellitus with other autoimmune disease:
    a. thyrotoxicosis
    b. Hashimoto's disease
    c. primary hypothyroidism
    d. idiopathic hypoparathyroidism
    e. idiopathic Addison's disease
    f. Schmidt's syndrome
    g. pernicious anemia
    h. myasthenia gravis
    i. polyendocrine disorders
4. Antibodies to other endocrine glands in juvenile onset diabetes mellitus
    a. thyroid
    b. adrenal
    c. gastric cells

controlling multiple serological expression of antigens, so called immune response genes which control the development of some mediated immunity to these antigens, may form the modality for carbohydrate intolerance expression in the diabetic syndrome. A summary of the possibility that diabetes is an autoimmune disease is depicted in Table 5.

Obesity

The problem of obesity is very closely intertwined with the entire diabetic syndrome. Approximately 80% of the adult onset diabetics are obese (Williams and Porte, 1974) and there are strong suggestions that control of the obesity would, to a large degree, erase the diabetes (Williams and Porte, 1974). Obesity is associated with hyperinsulinemia (Karam, Grodsky, and Forsham, 1963) and many individuals feel that the diabetes associated with obesity is, in actuality, an example of "high output" failure; however, most of these patients never advance to the degree of becoming ketoacidosis-prone diabetics. The studies of Barrett and Boshell (1962) called attention to the importance of a "tissue resistance" to insulin in the obese diabetic and this has been further defined by Roth (Archer *et al.*, 1975) who has demonstrated deficient insulin receptors in obesity. The importance of elevated basal hyperinsulinemia in obesity as a manifestation of resistance was pointed out by Porte (Bagdade, Bierman, and Porte, 1967) and Kriesberg (Kriesberg and Boshell, 1967). These investigators demonstrated that hyperinsulinemia exists in the chemical diabetic regardless of the degree of obesity and postprandial glucose level. This strongly supported a resistant factor in diabetes and emphasized the importance of extra-*beta* cell factors in diabetes. The studies of Kipnis (1970) did not agree with this concept; however, subsequently the findings of Tzagournis (Chiles and Tzagournis, 1970), Reaven (Reaven and Miller, 1968), and Danowski (Danowski, Morgan, Sunder, Moses, and Sabeh, 1967) have confirmed the presence of hyperinsulinemia in early diabetes.

TREATMENT

General Considerations

Now that the diabetes express is beginning to roll, there is great expectancy on the part of scientists and patients alike that major breakthroughs are just around the corner. We must, however, not forget the millions of patients who now have the disease and who may become the victim of one of the many complications of diabetes before the breakthroughs occur. In other words, "what do we do until the doctor comes?" Many individuals feel that we can't really do anything and, thus, do nothing and this attitude is actually supported, to some degree, by studies such as the University Group Diabetes Program. Actually, the results of this study caused us to reassess our entire approach to diabetes mellitus. Since the study concluded that oral agents were ineffective and perhaps toxic, one could certainly at the very best not feel that these drugs provided the answer. Many readers ignored the fact that even the Lente insulin, used in a single daily dose in this study, did not prevent the complications of diabetes and seemed little, if any, better than placebo. If one, therefore, returned to the drawing boards and somewhat to history, a few situations suggested another approach. First of all, during the Regular insulin era, 1926-32, there appeared to be fewer diabetic complications than at any other time in history (Johnson, 1960). One must admit that these data are retrospective and that they do not enjoy randomization, etc., that would please the statistician but perhaps therein lies at least a kernel of truth. Another factor that emerged is that the pills as used in the UGDP study and the single shot of intermediate-acting Lente insulin did not prevent the rather marked rises in blood glucose one and two hours after meals or after a specific glucose load. The administration of Regular insulin a few minutes prior to the meal or glucose load appears to more nearly simulate nature and prevent the extreme rises in glucose. Thus, if insulin deficiency and the resultant hyperglycemia provide a milieu for the development of the thickened capillary membranes and subsequent microangiopathy then, perhaps, we should concern ourselves with more adequate control of these factors throughout the 24-*hour* period. Somogyi (1959) called attention to the "brittleness" that is provoked by insulin reactions and hypoglycemia and urged the use of Regular insulin. Molnar (1971) documented the effectiveness of multiple doses of Regular insulin in improving control. Based on these findings, we have modified Somogyi's approach of doing hourly quantitative urine sugars and instead collect four pools per day, *i.e.*, bedtime to breakfast, breakfast to lunch, lunch to supper, and supper to bedtime and we modified Molnar's three shots of Regular insulin per day to a combination of NPH plus Regular insulin before breakfast and the same combination before supper. Occasionally in the very difficult patient three doses per day of Regular plus a small dose of NPH insulin prior to supper or at bedtime is used. We quantitate the glucose in each urine pool and teach the patient to adjust his insulin based on glycosuria and patterned blood sugars (Boshell, 1976). Control can be smoothed out and, hopefully, on this program complications will be less.

This is what we are doing clinically while trying scientifically to find a cure or better methods of control. Possible therapeutic approaches for the future include pancreatic transplantation; an artificial pancreas with sensor, computer, and pump; immunization against certain viruses; or possibly the production of tolerance (Figure 4).

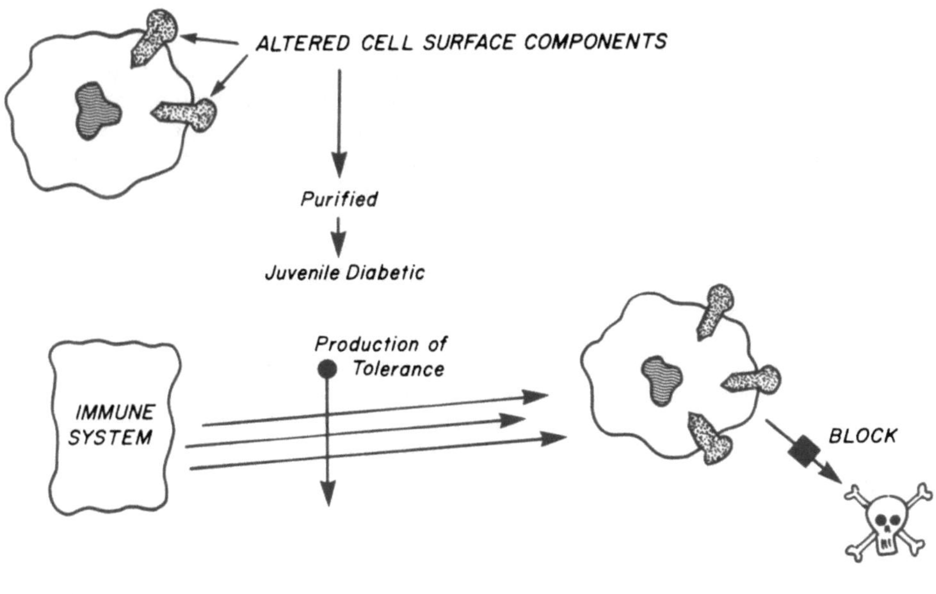

Figure 4. Possible therapeutic intervention by way of immune interference.

Pancreatic Transplantation

Organ transplantation was, to a large degree, initiated in this country with the successful transfer of a kidney between two closely related persons (Murray, Merrill, and Harrison, 1955). This has, of course, been extended now by the use of kidneys from human cadavers (Hume, 1968) and for a period of time from other primates (Hume, 1968). The dramatic heart transplant by Christian Barnard (1967) brought world wide attention to the transplant problem. Pancreatic transplants were actually performed with some degree of success as early as 1927 by Gayet (Gayet and Guillamie, 1927) and by Houssay (Houssay, 1929).

Because of the serious technical problems and complications of whole organ transplantation, attempts to refine the *beta* cell transplantation have been made with fragments of fetal pancreatic tissue (Browning and Resnick, 1951). The procedure above plus transplantation of isolated adult rat islets (Younoszai, Sorenson, and Lindall, 1970) has been moderately successful. The exocrine portion of the pancreatic fragments has presented some problem because of enzymatic autodigestion of the fragment or damage to the host. Fetal fragments, however, have very little exocrine function and a high percentage of islet tissue and, thus, have been used successfully (Leonard, Lazarow, McEvoy, and Hegre, 1974).

Pancreatic transplantation has been difficult, however, because of the fact that the surgeon must handle properly both the endocrine and exocrine pancreas. Not only blood flow but appropriate drainage for the exocrine pancreas must be established. Complications have consisted of vascular thrombosis, autodigestion, and graft rejection. Since 1966, 49 whole pancreas transplants in 47 recipients have been reported to the American College of Surgeons--National Institutes of Health Transplant Registry (Bergan, 1976). Only one of these individuals is alive with a functioning graft. In this patient and in three others surviving 10, 12, and 22 months, the metabolic deficiency of diabetes was relieved (ACS/NIH Organ Transplant Registry, 1971; Gliedman, Tellis, Soberman, Rifkin, Freed, and Veith, 1975).

If the *beta* cells can be encouraged to divide and grow *in vitro* and the problems of rejection can be conquered, there is good reason to think that banks of *beta* cells and other endocrine cells will be established and in widespread use in the not too distant future.

Artificial Pancreas

The first essential component of the artificial pancreas, the glucose sensor, was described by Hicks and Updike (1967). This was constructed by placing the glucose oxidase enzyme in a film of hydrogel over the teflon membrane covering a Clark (Clark and Sachs, 1968) oxygen probe, a platinum cathode. This approach was hampered because of the irreversible loss of enzyme activity. Modifications of this approach have been made by Bessman and Schultz (1973), by Soeldner (1975), and by Davis (1975).

The idea, of course, is to connect the glucose sensor to a miniaturized computer which will thus signal a delivery system to inject a certain amount of insulin into the circulation of the patient. Many problems in this area remain to be solved. How do you correct for an insulin overdose? How does one recalibrate to handle insulin resistance, etc." It is reasonable, however, to presume that solutions to the problems can be found and that clinical application of the "artificial pancreas" may be a reality within a few years. This will allow us to achieve more finite control in the insulin-dependent diabetic and provide a very useful tool in determining the effect of glucose control on diabetic complications (Albisser and Leibel, 1974). Pfeiffer (Pfeiffer, Thum, and Clemens, 1974) and investigators in Japan and Australia are currently evaluating working models of the artificial pancreas in animals. Additional miniaturization is necessary to make this clinically applicable.

Somatostatin

Somatostatin has provided another stimulus for the extra-pancreatic factors in diabetes, although studies now indicate that somatostatin-containing cells are also located in the pancreas (Orci, Baetens, Rufener, Amherdt, Ravazzola, Studer, Malaisse-Lagae, and Unger, 1976), as well as in the hypothalamus (Alpert, Brawer, Patel, and Reichlin, 1976). Somatostatin's major therapeutic role in diabetes would appear to be in its ability to inhibit the secretion of glucagon (Mortimer, Tunbridge, Carr, Yeomans, Lind, Coy, Bloom, Kastin, Mallison, Besser, Schally, and Hall, 1974). Unger (1971) has demonstrated that glucagon levels are abnormally high in diabetes. The studies of Gerich (Gerich, Lorenzi, Schneider, Karam, Rivier, Guillemin, and Forsham, 1974) have demonstrated a markedly ameliorative effect of somatostatin in insulin-dependent diabetic patients. If the problem of possible hematologic toxicity (del Guerico, di Natale, Gargantini, Garlaschi, and Chiumello, 1976) and short half-life (Besser, Mortimer, Carr, Schally, Coy, Evered, Kastin, Tunbridge, Thorner, and Hall, 1974) of somatostatin can be solved, this agent may become a very helpful tool in the management of diabetes. Somatostatin has been an eye-opener to the possible importance of the neuroendocrines in the diabetic syndrome.

A hyperactive sympathetic system, to a large degree, simulates diabetes and bits of evidence have accumulated to suggest that the neuroendocrine system may play a role in the etiology, the treatment, and the complications of diabetes mellitus. Pfeiffer (1965) and coworkers have described elevated growth hormone levels in prediabetes, while Müller (Müller, Faloona, Aguilar-Parada, and Unger, 1970) in Unger's laboratory pointed out the relatively high glucagon levels in diabetes. Overactive adrenergic receptors have been noted by Robertson (Robertson, Hazzard, Brunzell, Lerner, and Porte, 1972) and permanent diabetes has been produced in partially depancreatized dogs with catecholamine infusion by Loubatieres (Loubatiéres, Mariani, Chapal, and Rondot, 1964). There is much evidence to suggest a hypothalamic lipostat in obesity (Rabinowitz, 1970) and, since we have now gained some insight into hypothalamic control via the neurotransmitters, a therapeutic approach to obesity via chemical control of these centers may successfully control obesity and, hence, about 80% of the adult-onset diabetics.

COMPLICATIONS

The complications of diabetes may be logically divided into two broad categories--acute and chronic. The acute problems consist of hypoglycemia, ketoacidosis, hyperosmolar coma, and lactic acidosis. These are, to a large degree, preventable; the mechanism basically clear; and the therapy well understood.

On the other hand, the chronic complications, *i.e.*, retinopathy, neuropathy, nephropathy, and general cardiovascular abnormalities remain an enigma for the most part as to etiology and treatment. The chronic complications can be further subdivided into microvascular and macrovascular disease.

The work of Spiro (1971), Winegrad (Winegrad and Green, 1976), and others (Kilo, Vogler, and Williamson, 1972) suggest that the microvascular disease is, at least in part, caused by the insulin deficiency and resultant hyperglycemia of the diabetic syndrome. This is in contrast to the earlier suggestions of Siperstein (Siperstein *et al.*, 1966) that the early phases of microangiopathy actually preceded the carbohydrate abnormality. In the insulin-deficient hyperglycemic state the tissues that do not require insulin for glucose transport, *i.e.*, liver, brain, etc. (Gabbay, 1973), receive floods of glucose whereas the tissues that are insulin-dependent, *i.e.*, muscle, adipose tissue, etc. (Atkinson, 1971) are glucopenic. Furthermore, glucose pathways change quantitatively whereby the uridine diphosphate pathway (Spiro, 1971), sorbitol pathway (Gabbay, 1973), and hexose monophosphate shunt (Stewart, Sherman, and Anthony, 1966) become more active. The substrate for the formation of the capillary membrane increases (Kilo *et al.*, 1972) and the enzymes responsible for the process become more active thereby enhancing the formation of the glycoprotein membrane. Furthermore, the increased formation of sorbitol causes intracellular hyperosmolality when the glucose in the surrounding milieu decreases. Thus, for a period of time this pulls water into the cell causing disruption of the internal milieu and the formation of cataracts (van Heyningen, 1962) in the lens of the eye and possibly a depository site for lipids, platelets, etc. in the large vessel endothelium.

Low levels of 2,3-DPG are found in the hyperglycemic state (Alberti and Emerson, 1972). This shifts the oxygen dissociation curve to the left and may cause relative tissue anoxia (Kanter, Gerson, and Bessman, 1977). This may be the stimulus for new vessel proliferation which produces fragile capillaries in the eye and kidney with resultant easy bleeding and scarring.

The opportunity to determine just how important the hyperglycemia and other metabolic abnormalities associated with insulin deficiency are in the etiology of diabetic complications can be determined clinically only by a long-term prospective study with randomization of patients into close control and loose control protocols. A workable artificial pancreas and/or successful pancreatic transplantation will markedly enhance the possibility of accomplishing this.

One, of course, cannot ignore the importance of genetics in the vascular lesions of diabetes. This includes both microvascular and macrovascular diseases. The proposals of Benditt (Vracho and Benditt, 1974) are very stimulating in this regard. The input of the neuroendocrines into etiology, treatment, and complications is only beginning, but future investigation here will likely be very rewarding.

SUMMARY

The future in diabetic research is both stimulating and exciting. Diagnostic subclassification as to specific etiology appears well underway and will provide a more scientific basis for therapeutic approaches. The importance of the histocompatibility complex and its many secrets are rapidly becoming apparent in the etiology of juvenile diabetes. Further studies in obesity and the neuroendocrines may solve adult-onset diabetes. Pancreatic transplantation and artificial devices may provide important therapeutic approaches.

Further genetic explorations will, no doubt, provide clarity to the somewhat muddy picture of both etiology and complications. The challenges are here, let's hope that enough young scientists hear the call to provide the manpower to solve this major dilemma.

REFERENCES

ACS/NIH Organ Transplant Registry. 1971. First scientific report. *J. Amer. Med. Assoc.* **2**(7):1520-1529.

Alberti, K.G.M. and Emerson, P.E. 1972. 2,3-Diphosphoglycerate and tissue oxygenation in uncontrolled diabetes mellitus. *Lancet* **2**:391-395.

Alpert, L.C., Brawer, J.R., Patel, Y.C., and Reichlin, S. 1976. Somatostatinergic neurons in anterior hypothalamus: Immunohistochemical localization. *Endocrinology* **98**:255-258.

Albisser, A.M. and Leibel, B.S. 1974. Clinical control of diabetes by the artificial pancreas. *Diabetes* **23**:397-404.

Antoniades, H.M., Gundersen, K., Beigelman, P.M., Pyle, H.M., and Bougas, J.A. 1962. Studies on the state, transport, and regulation of insulin in human blood. *Diabetes* **11**:261-270.

Archer, J.A., Gordon, P., and Roth, J. 1975. Defect in insulin binding to receptors in obese man. Amelioration with calorie restriction. *J. Clin. Invest.* **55**:166-174.

Atkinson, D.E. 1971. p. 1. IN H.J. Vogel (Ed.) *Metabolic pathways.* Vol. V. New York: Academic Press.

Bach, F.H. and van Rood, J.J. 1976a. The major histocompatibility complex-genetics and biology. *New Eng. J. Med.* **295**:806-813.

Bach, F.H. and van Rood, J.J. 1976b. The major histocompatibility complex-genetics and biology. *New Eng. J. Med.* **295**:872-878.

Bach, F.H. and van Rood, J.J. 1976c. The major histocompatibility complex-genetics and biology. *New Eng. J. Med.* **295**:927-936.

Bagdade, J.D., Bierman, E.L., and Porte, D. Jr. 1967. The significance of basal insulin levels in the evaluation of the insulin response to glucose in diabetic and non-diabetic subjects. *J. Clin. Invest.* **46**:1549-1557.

Banting, F.G. and Best, C.H. 1922. The internal secretion of the pancreas. *J. Lab. Clin. Med.* **7**:251-266.

Barnard, C.N. 1967. A human cardiac transplant. *S. Afr. J. Med.* **41**:1271-1280.

Barret, J.C. and Boshell, B.R. 1962. Tolbutamide in the therapy of insulin resistance. *Diabetes* **11**:35-41.

Bennett, P.H., Burch, T.A., and Miller, M. 1971. Diabetes mellitus in American (Pima) Indians. *Lancet* **2**:125-128.

Bergan, J.J. 1976. *Amer. Coll. Surg./Nat'l. Inst. Health Organ Tranplant Registry Newsletter* **16**(April).

Besser, G.M., Mortimer, C.H., Carr, D., Schally, A.V., Coy, D.H., Evered, D., Kastin, A.J., Tunbridge, W.M.G., Thorner, M.O., and Hall, R. Growth hormone release-inhibiting hormone in acromegaly. *Br. Med. J.* **1**:352-355.

Bessman, S.P. and Schultz, R.D. 1973. Prototype glucose-oxygen sensor for the artificial pancreas. *Trans. Am. Soc. Artif. Intern. Organs* **19**:361-364.

Boshell, B.R. 1976. *Diabetes mellitus case studies.* Flushing, NY: Medical Examination Publishing Co., Inc.

Browning, H. and Resnick, P. 1951. Homologous and heterologous transplantation in pancreatic tissue in normal and diabetic mice. *Yale J. Biol. Med.* **24**:141-152.

Chandalia, H.B. and Boshell, B.R. 1970. Diagnosis of diabetes: The size and nature of the carbohydrate load. *Diabetes* **19**: 863-869.

Chiles, R. and Tzagournis, M. 1970. Excessive serum insulin response to oral glucose in obesity and mild diabetes. *Diabetes* **19**:458-464.

Clark, L.C. and Sachs, G. 1968. Bioelectrodes for tissue metabolism. *Ann. NY Acad. Sci.* **148**:133-153.

Cudworth, A.G. and Woodrow, J.C. 1975. HL-A system and diabetes mellitus. *Diabetes* **24**:345-349.

Danowski, T.S., Morgan, C.R., Sunder, J.H., Moses, C., and Sabeh, G. 1967. Immunoassayable insulin and glucose tolerance in non-obese and obese subjects. *Exp. Med. Surg.* **25**:122-130.

Davis, T.A. 1976. A laminated glucose sensor. Report of the National Commission on Diabetes to the Congress of the United States, submitted Dec. 10, 1975. III(3):316-317.

Gabbay, K.H. 1973. The sorbitol pathway and complications of diabetes. *New Eng. J. Med.* **288**:831-836.

Ganda, O.P. and Soeldner, S. 1977. Genetic, acquired, and related factors in the etiology of diabetes mellitus. *Arch. Intern. Med.* **137**:461-469.

Gayet, R. and Guillamie, M. 1927. La regulation de la secretion interne pancreatique par un processus humoral, demontree par des transplantations de pancreas. Experiences sur des animaux normaux. *C.R. Soc. Biol.* (Paris) **97**:1613-1614.

Gerich, J.E., Lorenzi, M., Schneider, V., Karam, J.H., Rivier, J., Guillemin, R., and Forsham, P.H. 1974. Effects of somatostatin on plasma glucose and glucagon levels in human diabetes mellitus - pathophysiologic and therapeutic implications. *New Eng. J. Med.* **291**:544-547.

Gliedman, M.L., Tellis, V., Soberman, R., Rifkin, H., Freed, S.Z., and Veith, F.J. 1975. The clinical use of steroids in pancreatic transplantation. *Transplant. Proc.* **7**:93-98.

Gottlieb, M.S. and Root, H.F. 1968. Diabetes mellitus in twins. *Diabetes* **17**:693-704.

del Guercio, M.H., di Natale, B., Gargantini, L., Garlaschi, C., and Chiumello, G. 1976. Effect of somatostatin on blood sugar plasma growth hormone, and glucagon levels in diabetic children. *Diabetes* **25**:550-553.

Hagedorn, H.C., Jensen, B.N., Krarup, N.B., and Wodstrup, I. 1936. Protamine insulate. *Acta Med. Scand.* **78**(Suppl.):678-684.

van Heyningen, R. 1962. The sorbitol pathway in the lens. *Exp. Eye Res.* **1**:396-404.

Hicks, G.P. and Updike, S.J. 1967. The enzyme electrode. *Nature* **214**:986-988.

Houssay, B.A. 1929. Technique de la greffe pancreaticoduodenale au cou. *C.R. Soc. Biol.* (Paris) **100**:138-140.

Houssay, B.A. 1937. Diabetes as a disturbance of endocrine regulation. *Am. J. Med. Sci.* **193**:581-606.

Hume, D.L. 1968. Kidney transplantation. IN F.L. Rapaport and J. Dausset (Eds.) *Human transplantation.* New York: Grune and Stratton.

Johnson, S. 1960. Retinopathy and nephropathy in diabetes mellitus: Comparison of the effects of two forms of treatment. *Diabetes* **9**:1-8.

Kanter, Y., Gerson, J.R., and Bessman, A.N. 1977. 2,3-Diphosphoglycerate, nucleotide phosphate, and organic and inorganic phosphate levels during the early phases of diabetic ketoacidosis. *Diabetes* **26**:429-433.

Karam, J.H., Grodsky, G.M., and Forsham, P.H. 1963. Excessive insulin response to glucose in obese subjects as measured by immunochemical assay. *J. Amer. Diab. Assn.* **12**:197-204.

Kilo, C., Vogler, N., and Williamson, J.R. 1972. Muscle capillary basement membrane changes related to aging and to diabetes mellitus. *Diabetes* **21**:881-905.

Kinoshita, J.H., Merola, L.O., Satoh, K., and Dikmak, E. 1962. Osmotic changes caused by the accumulation of dulcitol in lenses of rats fed with galactose. *Nature* **194**:1085-1087.

Kipnis, D.M. 1970. Insulin secretion in normal and diabetic individuals. *Adv. Intern. Med.* **16**:103-134.

Leonard, R.J., Lazarow, A., McEvoy, R.C. and Hegre, O. 1974. Islet cell transplantation. *Kidney Int.* **6**(Suppl. 1):S169-178.

Loubatières, A., Mariani, M.M., Chapal, J., and Rondot, A.M. 1964. Diabète sucré provoqué chez le chien par perfusion tempoaire d'adrenaline dans l'artere pancréatico-duodénale. *C.R. Soc. Biol.* (Paris) **158**:1688-1691.

Matschinsky, F.M., Landgraf, R., Ellerman, J., and Kotler-Brajtburg, J. 1972. Glucoreceptor mechanisms in islets of Langerhans. *Diabetes* **21** (Suppl. 2):555-569.

Mimura, G. 1971. Epidemiology of diabetes in Asia. pp. 331-344. IN R.R. Rodriquez and J. Vallance-Owen (Eds.) *Diabetes.* Amsterdam: Excerpta Medica.

Molnar, G.D. 1971. Clinical use of various insulin preparations. p. 139. IN S.S. Fajans and K.E. Sussman (Eds.) *Diabetes mellitus: Diagnosis and treatment.* Vol. III. New York: American Diabetes Assn., Inc.

Mortimer, C.H., Tunbridge, W.M., Carr, D., Yeomans, L., Lind, T., Coy, D.H., Bloom, S.R., Kastin, A., Mallinson, C.N., Besser, G.M., Schally, A.V., and Hall, R. 1974. Effects of growth-hormone release inhibiting hormone on circulating glucagon, insulin, and growth hormone in normal, diabetic, acromegalic, and hypopituitary patients. *Lancet* **1**:697-701.

Müller, W.A., Faloona, G.R., Aguilar-Parada, E., and Unger, R.H. 1970. Abnormal *alpha*-cell function in diabetes response to carbohydrate and protein ingestion. *New Eng. J. Med.* **283**: 109-115.

Murray, J.E., Merrill, J.P., and Harrison, J.H. 1955. Renal related homotransplantation in identical twins. *Surg. Forum* **6**:432-438.

O'Brien, D. 1970. Evidence for an abnormal insulin in diabetes mellitus. *Acta Diabetol. Lat.* **7**:211-219.

Orci, L., Baetens, D., Rufener, C., Amherdt, M., Ravazzola, M., Studer, P., Malaisse-Lagae, F., and Unger, R.H. 1976. Hypertrophy and hyperplasia of somatostatin-containing D-cells in diabetes. *Proc. Nat'l. Acad. Sci.* USA **73**:1338-1342.

Pfeiffer, E.F. 1965. Recognized diabetogenic hormones and diabetes in man. p. 368. IN *On the nature and treatment of diabetes*. Amsterdam: Excerpta Medica.

Pfeiffer, E.F., Thum, C., and Clemens, A.H. 1974. The artificial *beta* cell--a continuous control of blood sugar by external regulation of insulin infusion. *Horm. Metab. Res.* **6**:339-342.

Rabinowitz, D. 1970. Some endocrine and metabolic aspects of obesity. *Ann. Rev. Med.* **21**:241-258.

Reaven, G.M. and Miller, R. 1968. Study of the relationship between glucose and insulin responses to an oral glucose load in man. *Diabetes* **17**:560-569.

Report of the National Commission on Diabetes to the Congress of the United States. Submitted December 10, 1975.

Rifkin, H. 1962. Current concepts of diabetic microangiopathy. *Adv. Intern. Med.* **11**:235-272.

Robertson, R.B., Hazzard, W.R., Brunzell, W.R., Lerner, R.L., and Porte, D. 1972. Paradoxical hypoinsulinemia: An *alpha*-adrenergic mediated response to glucose. *Lancet* **2**:787-789.

Sanger, F. 1959. Chemistry of insulin. *Science* **129**:1340-1344.

Siperstein, M.D. 1976. The glucose tolerance test: A pitfall in the diagnosis of diabetes mellitus. *Adv. Int. Med.* **20**:297-323.

Siperstein, M.D., Norton, W., Unger, R.H., and Madison, L.L. 1966. Muscle capillary basement membrane within normal, diabetic, and prediabetic patients. *Trans. Assn. Am. Physicians* **79**:330-347.

Soeldner, J.S. 1975. The glucose monitor-artificial *beta* cell program. Report of the National Commission on Diabetes to the Congress of the United States, III(3):327-331.

Somogyi, M. 1959. Exacerbation of diabetes by excess insulin action. *Am. J. Med.* **26**:169-191.

Spiro, R.G. 1963. Glycoproteins and diabetes. *J. Am. Diet. Assn.* **12**:223-230.

Spiro, R.G. 1971. Biochemical basis of diabetic microangiopathy. pp. 275-280. IN S.S. Fajans and K.E. Sussman (Eds.) *Diabetes mellitus: Diagnosis and treatment*. Vol. III. New York: American Diabetes Assn., Inc.

Steiner, D.F., Cunningham, D., Spigelman, L., and Aten, B. 1967. Insulin biosynthesis: Evidence for a precursor. *Science* **157**:697-700.

Stewart, W.A., Sherman, W.R., and Anthony, S. 1966. Free sugars in alloxan diabetic rat nerve. *Biochem. Biophys. Res. Commun.* 22:488-491.

Sutherland, E.W. and Rall, T.W. 1958. Fractionation and characterization of a cyclic adenine ribonucleotide formed by tissue particles. *J. Biol. Chem.* 232:1077-1091.

Tattersall, R.B. and Pyke, D.A. 1972. Diabetes in identical twins. *Lancet* 2:1120-1125.

Unger, R.H. and Madison, L.R. 1958. A new diagnostic procedure for mild diabetes mellitus: Evaluation of an intravenous tolbutamide response test. *Diabetes* 7:455-461.

Vallance-Owen, J. 1964. Synalbumin insulin antagonism. *Diabetes* 13:241-246.

Vracho, R. and Benditt, E.P. 1974. Manifestations of diabetes mellitus: Their possible relationship to an underlying cell defect. *Am. J. Path.* 75:204-221.

White, P. and Graham, C.A. 1971. The child with diabetes. pp. 339-360. IN A. Marble, P. White, R.F. Bradley, and L.P. Krall (Eds.) *Joslin's diabetes mellitus.* Philadelphia: Lea and Febiger.

Wilkerson, H.L.C., Hyman, H., Kaufman, M., McCuistion, A.C., and Francis, J. O'S. 1960. Diagnostic evaluation of oral glucose tolerance tests in non-diabetic subjects after various levels of carbohydrate intake. *New Eng. J. Med.* 262:1047-1053.

Williams, R.H. and Porte, D., Jr. 1974. The pancreas. pp. 502-626. IN R.H. Williams (Ed.) *Textbook of endocrinology.* Philadelphia: W.B. Saunders Co.

Winegrad, A.I. 1972. Diabetic neuropathy. *New Eng. J. Med.* 286:1261-1262.

Winegrad, A.I. and Green, D.A. 1976. Diabetic polyneuropathy: The importance of insulin deficiency, hyperglycemia, and alterations of myoinositol metabolism in its pathogenesis. *New Eng. J. Med.* 295:1416-1421.

Yalow, R.S. and Berson, S.A. 1959. Assay of plasma insulin in human subjects by immunological methods. *Nature* 184 (Suppl. 21):1648-1649.

Yalow, R.S. and Berson, S.A. 1960. Immunoassay of endogenous plasma insulin in man. *J. Clin. Invest.* 39:1156-1175.

Younoszai, R., Sorenson, R.L., and Lindall, A.W. 1970. Homotransplantation of isolated pancreatic islets. *Diabetes* 19 (Suppl. 1): 406. (Abstr.)

DISCUSSION FOLLOWING DR. BOSHELL'S TALK

Dr. Jackson

Thank you, Dr. Boshell, for your comprehensive and informative presentation. To open the discussion, I would like to ask Dr. Charles Kilo, because of his extensive clinical experience, to make a few remarks.

Dr. Kilo

I have enjoyed the excellent presentations made at this outstanding symposium in honor of Dr. Jackson. He has been a pioneer leader in advancing the need for good blood sugar control.

I concur with the remarks made by Dr. Boshell. He stressed the tremendous need for increased financial resources and for improved patient care and management. The rate of increase in the incidence of diabetes is epidemic and a major national health problem. We must, therefore, encourage many more physicians to specialize in diabetes research and in the care and management of the diabetic patient.

Dr. Breitenbach

Dr. Boshell, you presented evidence on the effects of testosterone, glucocorticoids, and stress, all of which are lympholytic and would be affecting or modifying, in one way or another, the immune response and would have implications on the HLA antigen. Is there any evidence of a T-cell deficiency or any other deficiency in juvenile diabetics?

Dr. Boshell

Dr. Forsham, some years ago, studied cortisol and adrenal function in the diabetic. Although there are documented abnormalities in glucagon and growth hormone, we don't have good evidence that steroids play an important role etiologically. I'm not sure that the immune response in diabetics has been studied extensively enough to answer your question.

Dr. Peterson

I wonder if you have any insights into the effects of diabetes or hyperglycemia on the hypothalamic-pituitary-gonadal axis?

Dr. Boshell

Our observations and clinical studies show that female diabetics in poor control frequently have disturbances in menstrual function and problems with fertility, whereas those who are in good control have not had such problems unless they were obese. I have seen many men under 50 who have developed impotence. Some studies have shown decreased spermatogenesis in some of these men, mostly in those whose diabetes was not particularly well controlled. I don't know of any elaborate studies in terms of pituitary-hypothalamic function. We feel that there is a tremendous amount of exploration that should be done in this area and now are recruiting a full-time investigator in neuroendocrinology.

Dr. Burns

I wanted to ask you, Dr. Boshell, how you characterized this well-controlled group that has, thus far, not had any complications, in terms of biochemical markers, blood sugars, or urine sugars? Are you looking at hemoglobin A_{Ic} and has that been helpful in putting them into one group or another?

Dr. Boshell

We have a group that is starting to measure A_{Ic}. I would hope that it might be helpful but I'm a little dubious that it's going to be nearly as helpful as we'd like for it to be. As to assessing control, we have our patients make fractional urine collections. We try to have them spill no more than 4 *g* of glucose in a single pool and, hopefully, much less. We try to prevent frequent insulin reactions, and we don't see a lot of severe insulin reactions. We standardize the diet and try to keep that stable and we teach them to change their insulin to take care of the other variables. They take at least two doses of insulin daily, part of it NPH and part of it regular insulin, before breakfast and again before supper. If they are extremely labile, they're on three doses of regular insulin a day with a small amount of NPH insulin added before the evening meal. We teach them that, when they're having a lot of trouble, they should check the quantitative pooled urine using the Clinitest two-drop method, provided that we've established that their renal threshold is fairly normal. We use this method more than the blood sugar. If the renal threshold's high, we resort to teaching them to measure their blood sugar with Dextrostix. We strive to maintain all of the blood sugars under 150 *mg/dℓ* without a significant number of insulin reactions.

Dr. Sanny

Are there any problems, social or economic, in which patients will not seek medical help due to finances, and are there any ways in which the clinics are helping the less fortunate patients?

Dr. Boshell

Since we raised the money for our hospital from the private sector, we never turn a patient away because of insufficient funds. We will see them, give them outpatient care, and the whole teaching program even if they can't afford to pay.

We can't do that on an inpatient basis because we're part of the university system and we don't have the funds to support that. However, with a total team setup, you can cut the costs for all patients fantastically by keeping them out of the hospital.

Dr. Jackson

I have been asked by Dr. Boshell to share with you my recommendations concerning the management of children with juvenile diabetes. Before doing that, I would like to take this opportunity to thank all of you who have made this conference possible, especially Dr. Calvin Woodruff and Dr. David Klachko, who were primarily responsible for arranging the program. I deeply appreciate all of the kind remarks made during this meeting regarding my contribution to improve the care of children with insulin-dependent diabetes. To conclude the meeting, let us focus our attention on the child with diabetes.

Most physicians recognize the necessity of knowing how to treat the life-threatening complications of diabetes. However, the difficulties encountered in the long-term treatment of diabetes in the child are so numerous that too often the disease is managed inadequately. Many internists and ophthalmologists have become convinced that a higher degree of control is desirable in an attempt to delay, or prevent, the vascular changes. On the other hand, many pediatricians and family physicians remain skeptical. Those who treat only a few diabetic children do not see the insidious development of complications. In the child, vascular changes develop slowly over many years and are not detectable clinically until early- or mid-adult life.

In my opinion, most children with overt diabetes receive delayed and inadequate treatment at the time of onset of symptoms. Too often the children are managed as if they were small adults. If the diagnosis is made before the onset of ketoacidosis, precious time may be lost by observing the response of the child to nothing more than a modified dietary plan. After a few days, when the dietary management is found ineffective, some of the children are then submitted to an ineffective therapeutic trial with an oral hypoglycemic agent--even though many studies indicate that oral hypoglycemic agents are not effective for the treatment of children with overt diabetes. At that time, once-daily doses of an intermediate-type insulin are usually prescribed. Because most diabetic children continue to produce varying amounts of endogenous insulin during the early weeks, or even months, after onset of overt disease, they will have a good response to an improved diet and once-daily injections of insulin. Nevertheless, we have found that to approximate physiological control closely, patients need carefully structured meal plans and at least twice-daily injections of insulin. Our experience indicates that in those who receive suboptimal treatment with insulin given only once daily, the insulin deficiency gradually progresses.

Diabetes in children and young adults is so different from diabetes in the middle-aged or elderly that it requires special consideration. Every child with overt diabetes should receive insulin therapy as soon as the diagnosis is confirmed. The earlier the diagnosis is made, the lower the amount of insulin needed and the easier it will be to attain and maintain a high degree of control with little risk of hypoglycemia. There is growing evidence that the glucose tolerance test of children, as well as of adults, may be abnormal (chemical diabetes) for years before the onset of clinical, or overt, diabetes. Studies of children with a family history of diabetes during intercurrent infections or during their growth spurt verify the desirability of doing oral glucose tolerance tests to detect diabetes in the preclinical state.

A child with recent onset of overt diabetes should be hospitalized as soon as possible in a medical center with a staff experienced in management of children with diabetes, to replete the nutritional state and determine the maintenance insulin requirement. Duration of hospitalization varies, depending on how early the diagnosis is made; but average time is usually three to five weeks. A school program and recreational outlets should be available so that the child may continue his education and have supervised physical activity, not only for his overall well-being but also to make it possible to regulate the daily insulin dosage.

In addition to medical care, the child and family need intensive and continuous education from a nurse and dietitian experienced in the management of children with diabetes. The educators need to spend considerable time with the child and parents, both in the hospital and when the child and parents return to the clinic for periodic visits. It is necessary and important to instruct both parents and have each participate in the care of the child. The physician should use all facilities and personnel available to him in evaluating and educating the family. Ideally, the physician, nurse, dietitian, and social worker should meet with the family as a team. Each member of that team can provide unique expertise on some aspect of the management of diabetes mellitus. Not only the family but often the community needs to be educated if the patient is to make a good adjustment. The time to undertake a detailed social evaluation of the family is during the initial hospitalization, as the ultimate prognosis will be directly related to the socioeconomic condition of the child's family. The easiest time to attain compliance is at the onset of the disease. Although the child should gradually assume more responsibility for his own care, it is undesirable and unrealistic to expect children or adolescents to assume primary responsibility for that care.

The maintenance diet for the child with diabetes should be essentially the same as that for normal children. For that reason, we generally avoid the word "diet" in talking to patients and their parents. "Diet" has a connotation of fasting and denial; "meal plan" does not. The meal plan for the child with diabetes should be based on the nutritional needs of healthy, nondiabetic children of similar age, height, and weight and should be compatible with the family's income and food habits. The essential difference is that food intake for the diabetic child is adjusted to the type and dose of insulin given and to his pattern of physical activity. The child's family needs to understand that the patient's meal plan is reasonable for all members of the family. One of the most effective ways for the family to help the child is to establish regularity in meal patterns, to avoid the use of poor quality foods, and to adopt the same basic food plan advocated for the patient.

Physical activity and its relation to insulin and food intake are also important aspects of diabetic management. The well-controlled diabetic child may be as active as any child with whom he plays. It is not necessary to limit physical activity; it is, however, necessary to understand his needs for more or less food, depending on variations in that activity.

There is no doubt that the child's diabetes imposes an emotional stress on both the child and his family. In our opinion, it is a cruel delusion that proper control of the disease can be attained only at the expense of emotional health. On the contrary, it is our experience and the opinion of others that the self-discipline upon which proper control depends actually can serve to make the patient psychologically better adjusted.

Current knowledge makes possible good control of diabetics, which can delay or prevent the insidious development of progressive vascular disease. Recent advances in diabetes research are encouraging. We are looking forward to the day when we will know the cause of diabetes and how to prevent it. Until then, we need to develop resources to better apply current knowledge.

SUBJECT INDEX

Acanthosis nigricans, 94, 96-98
    type B patients, 98, 101-102
Acetylcholine, 12, 37, 39, 70-71, 98
Adenyl cyclase, 40
Adipocyte, 102-103
Alloxan, 68, 71, 80, 107, 109, 128, 147
α-adrenergic agonist, 37, 56
β-adrenergic agonist, 37, 56
Adrenergic blockade, 38
Alpha (α,A) cells, 6, 12, 22-23, 31, 37, 55, 57, 60-61, 63-64, 66-67, 71, 73
Amino acid, 26, 30-31, 34, 39-41, 112, 147, 149, 150-152, 176
    alanine, 35-36
    arginine, 35, 42, 60-61, 69-71
    asparagine, 106, 143
    aspartic acid, 143
    glycine, 142, 144
    half-cystine, 142-144
    hydroxylysine, 106-107, 142-144, 146-152
    hydroxyproline, 142, 150-152
    leucine, 69-70
    lysine, 106-107, 143, 146, 148-149
    proline, 149-151
    tyrosine, 143-144
    valine, 144
Amylase, 3
Antibodies, 168, 178
    anti-DNA, 96
    anti-insulin, 16, 21-22, 87, 89, 98
Antibodies, cont.
    anti-nuclear, 96
    anti-receptor, 96-98, 101-103
    auto-, 97
    gene, 177
Antisera, 30-31, 64
    antiglucagon, 31, 64
    antiinsulin, 64, 87, 147
    antisomatostatin, 64-65, 71-72
Atropine, 37

Basement membrane
    capillary, 133-138, 169
    glomerular, 106-107, 124, 141-153, 163, 167
Beta (β,B) cells, 6-7, 12, 15-18, 21-26, 57-58, 63-64, 66-67, 71, 73, 86, 102, 172, 177, 180-182, 184, 186
Beta-hydroxy butyric acid, 4

Calcium, 39, 58, 126-127
Catecholamine, 37, 188
Chylomicronemia, 35
Collagen, 106, 108, 133, 142-144, 146, 149, 150, 152
Coma, 4, 121
Complement (C_3), 168
Converting enzyme, 26
C-peptide, 15-18, 21-27, 60, 130
Cyclic AMP (c-AMP), 40, 59, 69-70, 176

Delta (D) cells, 11, 63-64, 66-68, 70-73
Depancreatized, 5, 188
Diabetes insipidus, 1
Diabetes mellitus
adult onset, 3, 24, 83, 162-163, 177-180, 182-183, 188-189
maturity onset, 43, 135
obese diabetes, 3-4, 12-13, 24
onset, 3, 16, 22, 43, 56-57, 60, 68, 103, 129, 135-136, 177-179, 180, 182-183
overt, 25, 103-104, 129, 133, 170-171, 179, 197-198
Dogs, 4, 35, 58, 71, 160, 188
canine, 36, 68, 70
Dopamine, 39

Endocrine glands
parathyroid, 80
thyroid, 80
Enzymes, 26, 125
aldose reductase, 109-112
beta-glycosidase, 152
CDP-diglyceride-inositol transferase, 116
collagenase, 138
galactosyltransferase, 148
glucose oxidase, 187
glucosyltransferase, 107-108, 124
glutamic decarboxylase, 12
glycosyltransferases, 141, 147-149
liver phosphorylase, 40
lysyl hydroxylase, 148
peptidases, 83
sorbitol dehydrogenase, 109
sugar transferase, 143
Epidermal growth factor, 7
Epinephrine, 37-39, 55-56, 70-71
Erythrocyte, 108-109, 125-126

Fatty acids, 39
Fetus, 41
fetal, 67
Free fatty acids (FFA), 35, 40, 55
Fundus A cells, 54

Galactose, 106, 111, 125
Gamma-aminobutyric acid (GABA), 6, 11-12
Gamma (γ) globulin, 31, 96
Gastric, 53-54, 65, 79
gastrin, 39, 54-55, 65, 70
gastric juice, 54
Gastric inhibitory polypeptide (GIP), 65, 70
Glomerulus, 106, 124, 138, 144-145, 158, 162-163
glomerulopathy, 157-158, 161-163
glomerulosclerosis, 106-107, 163
Glucagon (pancreatic), 6-7, 11-12, 17-18, 22-23, 27, 29-45, 53-61, 63, 65-66, 69-73, 82-84, 187-188, 195
Glucocorticoid, 38-39
Gluconeogenesis, 40-41, 44, 151
Gluconeogenic, 35
Glucose, 2, 6, 13, 18, 21-23, 29-30, 32-36, 38-45, 53, 55-56, 59, 69, 71-73, 81-82, 87-90, 95, 96, 101-103, 106, 136, 142-144, 148, 151-152, 157-158, 160, 169, 177, 180, 184-189, 196
Glucose tolerance test, 25, 33, 54, 58-59, 87, 96, 101-102, 158, 177, 198
Glutathione, 125
Glycogenolysis, 40-41
Glycosuria, 1, 4-5, 129, 167, 185
Golgi apparatus, 15
Granules, 15, 26, 67
Growth hormone, 7, 38-39, 42, 57-58, 65-66, 71, 80, 83, 195
Gut, 53, 65, 69, 71, 73

Hemoglobin, 105, 109
A_I, 18
A_{Ia}, 130
A_{Ib}, 130
A_{Ic}, 108-109, 128-129, 196
F, 109
Hepatic, 43-45
Homeostasis, 44, 61, 63
glucose homeostasis, 61, 73, 81, 90, 142
Hormones
ACTH, 65
calcitonin, 80
parathyroid hormone, 80
prolactin, 65
thyrotropin (TSH), 65, 71, 81, 98
triiodothyronine (T_3), 81
Hyperglucagonemia, 31, 36, 42, 44, 56, 59, 60
Hyperglycemia, 3, 6, 12-13, 23-24, 27, 29, 34-35, 41-42, 44, 56, 60-61, 82, 84, 102, 114, 117, 141, 147, 151-152, 167, 173, 184, 188-189, 195
Hyperglycemic-glycogenolytic factor (HGF), 6
Hyperinsulinemia, 12, 59, 68, 92-94, 96, 101, 183-184
Hypertension
Goldblatt, 163
Hypertriglyceridemia, 36
Hypoglycemia, 6, 22-23, 34, 38-39, 41, 60-61, 84, 101, 185, 188, 197-198
Hypoinsulinemia, 58-59
Hypoglucagonemia, 58
Hypothalamus, 11, 65, 71, 82, 92, 188
hypothalamic factor, 11, 65, 171
hypothalamic function, 196
LRH, 79
TRH, 79

Immunoglobulin, 97, 102, 158, 160-161, 163
IgG, 162, 167
IgM, 168

Inhibitors
of aldose reductase, 111
of cellular metabolism, 70
of collagenase alpha-1-antitrypsin, 138
alpha-2-macroglobulin, 138
of protease, 151
Insulin, 5-7, 11-13, 15-17, 21-27, 30-31, 34-35, 37, 39-44, 53-61, 63, 65-66, 70-73, 79, 81-98, 101-103, 105, 138, 141, 147, 152, 157-158, 160-163, 168, 173, 176, 180, 182-185, 187-188, 196-199
α-chain, 26
β-chain, 26
Insulin antibodies, 22
anti-insulin antiserum, 40, 64, 87, 147
Islets of Langerhans, 4-5, 13, 31, 58, 79
islets, 12, 63, 65-67, 69, 72-73, 80, 82, 101, 124, 158, 160, 180, 183, 186
Isoproterenol, 69-71

Ketoacidosis, 30-31, 42-43, 57, 121, 179-180, 183, 188, 197
ketosis, 42, 167
Ketogenesis, 40
Ketone bodies, 42, 55
Ketonemia, 29, 41
Ketosis, 42
Kidneys, 2, 81, 107, 124, 126, 134, 142, 144-149, 151-152, 158, 161-163, 167-168, 172-173, 186, 189
nephrectomy, 161-162
nephropathy, 142-143, 146-147, 152, 158, 160, 188
renal abnormalities, 113
renal disease, 142
renal failure, 31, 59
renal function, 113, 162
renal homografts, 172
renal threshold, 196
uninephrectomy, 196

L-dopa, 37
Leukocyte, 109, 138
Liver, 2, 3, 59, 90, 92, 108, 151, 188
  hepatic, 30, 40, 43-45, 108
Lymphocyte, 92, 95, 97

Mannoheptulose, 70-71
Mesangial, 160
  mesangial matrix, 158
  mesangium, 158, 163, 168
Microangiopathy, 160-161, 163-164, 167-168, 185, 188
Monocyte, 90-97, 101-102
Motilin, 65
Myasthenia gravis, 98
Myoinositol, 105, 110-117, 121-124, 126-128
Mystromys albicaudatus, 167

Neurotensin, 39
Norepinephrine, 39
Normoglycemia, 6, 103
  euglycemia, 26, 35

Obese, 3-4, 12-13, 24, 68, 89, 90-97, 167, 183-184
  nonobese, 101
  obese mice, 68, 95
  obesity, 7, 89, 90, 92-93, 95, 98, 175, 179, 183, 188
Opiates, 3
Oxygen, 109, 125
  oxygenate, 109
  oxygen diffusion, 112
  oxygen dissociation curve, 189
  oxygen transport, 164
  oxygen uptake, 112

Pancreas, 2-5, 11, 35-36, 42, 53, 57-58, 68, 70-71, 83, 172-173, 175, 185-187, 189
  canine, 32-33, 68
  human fetal, 67
Pancreas, cont.
  pancreatic, 1, 3, 7, 11-12, 17, 31-32, 63-64, 66, 68, 88
  pancreatic duct, 172
Pancreatectomy, 4, 30, 42, 56, 57
Pancreatic polypeptide, 6-7, 11, 63, 65
Parasympathetic, 37-39
Phentolamine, 38
Phlorhizin, 4
Placenta, 41
Plasma membrane, 86
Polyethylene glycol, 16, 22
Polyol, 105, 109-113, 117
Polyuria, 2
Postprandial, 25
Potassium, 110
Preproinsulin, 15
Proinsulin, 15-16, 21, 26-27, 82, 87, 89, 176
Propranolol, 38
Prostaglandin, 39, 57
Proteinuria, 96, 138, 142, 146, 152

Rabbits, 4, 41
Radioimmunoassay, 21, 30, 65, 89, 130, 161, 176
Rat, 40-41, 58, 67-68, 72, 122, 128, 148-152, 157-158, 160-161, 163, 168
  uremic rats, 59
Receptors, 178, 180
  acetylcholine, 98
  α-adrenergic, 37, 188
  α-cell glucoreceptor, 60-61
  β-adrenergic, 37, 188
  glucagon, 58-59
  glucose, 177
  insulin, 13, 59, 85-87, 90-98, 102-103, 175, 177, 182, 184
  TSH, 98
Renin, 65, 81
Retinopathy, 160-161, 188
Rough endoplasmic reticulum, 15
  endoplasmic reticulum, 110

Satiety, 26
Secretion, 6, 39, 65, 70
Serotonin, 6, 11-12, 37, 39, 63
Sheep, 41
  lamb, 56
Sodium, 110, 127
Somatostatin (SRIF), 6-7, 11-12, 30, 39, 41, 43-44, 53-56, 58-59, 63-73, 79-84, 175, 187
Sorbitol, 109, 112, 175, 188-189
Splanchnic, 53, 65, 80
Stains
  aldehyde fuchsin-trichrome, 64
  chrome-hematoxylin-phloxin, 64
  Heidenhains azan, 64
  phosphotungstic acid-hematoxylin, 64
  silver impregnation (Hellman-Hellerstrom), 64
Streptozotocin, 68, 107, 116, 124, 128, 147-149, 157, 168-169
Sympathetic, 38-39

Theophylline, 69-70
Tumor, 66, 68, 71-73

Urine, 1-2, 114, 185, 196
  uric acid, 3

Vagotomized, 37
Vagus nerve, 37
Vasoactive intestinal peptide, 63, 65

Xylose, 65, 81

MIX
Papier aus verantwortungsvollen Quellen
Paper from responsible sources
FSC® C105338

If you have any concerns about our products,
you can contact us on
ProductSafety@springernature.com

In case Publisher is established outside the EU,
the EU authorized representative is:
Springer Nature Customer Service Center GmbH
Europaplatz 3, 69115 Heidelberg, Germany

Printed by Libri Plureos GmbH
in Hamburg, Germany